THE
GASTROINTESTINAL
SOURCEBOOK

Other books by M. Sara Rosenthal

□ □ □

The Thyroid Sourcebook 2d ed.
The Gynecological Sourcebook 2d ed.
The Pregnancy Sourcebook 2d ed.
The Fertility Sourcebook
The Breastfeeding Sourcebook
The Breast Sourcebook

THE
GASTROINTESTINAL
SOURCEBOOK

◨ ◨ ◨

by M. Sara Rosenthal

Medical Adviser: Gary May, M.D., F.R.C.P.
Clinical Assistant Professor of Medicine,
Department of Medicine, Division of Gastroenterology,
University of Calgary

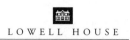

LOWELL HOUSE
LOS ANGELES
NTC/Contemporary Publishing Group

Although every effort has been made to ensure that the information provided here is accurate and up to date at the time of publication, this book is in no way intended to replace the advice of qualified health care professionals.

Library of Congress Cataloging in Publication Data
Rosenthal, M. Sara.
    The gastrointestinal sourcebook / by Sara M. Rosenthal
      p. cm.
    Includes bibliographical references and index.
    ISBN 1-56565-854-X
    ISBN 0-7373-0081-7 (paper)
    1. Gastrointestinal system—Diseases—Popular works. I. Title.
RC806.ZR67 1997
616.3'3—dc21   97-42116
                                                         CIP

Published by Lowell House, a division of NTC/Contemporary Publishing Group, Inc., 4255 West Touhy Avenue, Lincolnwood, Illinois 60646-1975 U.S.A.

Design by Carolyn Wendt
Illustration on page 3 by Elizabeth Weadon Massari

Printed and bound in the United States of America
International Standard Book Number: 0-7373-0081-7
10 9 8 7 6 5 4 3 2 1

To my husband . . . who says I give him heartburn.

CONTENTS

CONTENTS

ACKNOWLEDGMENTS

If it weren't for the commitment, hard work, and guidance of the following people, this book would never have been written:

Gary May, M.D., F.R.C.P., Clinical Assistant Professor of Medicine, Department of Medicine, Division of Gastroenterology, University of Calgary, bravely took on the task of acting as medical adviser for this book. His thoughtful comments and practical approach to gastroenterology is reflected throughout this book. Gillian Arsenault, M.D., M.HSc., F.R.C.P., continuously passed along important articles and "tidbits" that are part of this work. A special thank-you to Janssen-Ortho, Inc., who exposed me to a wealth of hard-to-find resources and experts on GI disorders.

As for my editorial team, Larissa Kostoff is the best editorial assistant I could have hoped for. Bud Sperry, my editor at Lowell House, and Maria Magallanes, managing editor at Lowell House, longtime comrades, are always supportive and very accommodating.

Finally, two special colleagues and friends, Janine Falcon and Gina Hudel, deserve a sincere: "thanks for putting up with me!" They are always there to listen to passages of text and seem to know when it's time to drag me away from my computer into civilization.

INTRODUCTION
Why GI?

The fastest path to wellness is through the stomach. According to the Ayurveda, an ancient Indian approach to holistic health, indigestion or incomplete digestion is the root of all illness. After having completed this book, I believe that's probably true.

It's not possible to research any health topic without accumulating a wealth of material on the digestive tract and general gastrointestinal (GI) problems. When I specifically researched GI disorders as an entity, I was shocked to discover how many people are affected by chronic upper GI symptoms, such as gastroesophageal reflux disease (GERD), as well as lower GI disorders ranging from irritable bowel syndrome to ulcerative colitis. Despite this, surprisingly little material is available to the layperson on GI disorders as a group of diseases, although there are libraries full of books on diet, nutrition, food, and so on. Most books on GI disorders focus on specific diseases, such as ulcerative colitis or Crohn's disease, but there is virtually nothing available on upper GI problems, nor on the GI tract as a whole. As many gastroenterologists (GI specialists) have told me, lower and upper GI symptoms often run together. For myself, understanding the universe of the digestive tract—a universe of digestive enzymes, muscles, nerves, and hormones—led me to truly understand many of my own GI symptoms. Like many people, I had come to accept them as normal. But being armed with the knowledge of how things truly work can make it easier for us to change our eating and life-style habits. The more I read, the more I began to see that persistent GI symptoms, however mild, are the body's way of telling us something's wrong. Food choices, timing of eating, gravity, stress, and sedentary life-styles can all affect our digestion. The more we ignore our digestive symptoms, the more unhealthy our bodies can become.

We are living amid an epidemic of digestive upset in the Western world. It's no accident that commercials during the national evening news are one of the best vehicles to sell stomach medications. If the news isn't enough to give you heartburn, then perhaps the fast food you "nuked" for dinner, which you're eating while watching the news, will do the trick. Despite the explosion in low-fat foods, we're getting fatter. At least 35 percent of North American men and 27 percent of North American women are obese, meaning that they weigh at least 20 percent more than the ideal weight for their age and height. We all know that obesity can put us at risk for cardiovascular problems or Type II diabetes (noninsulin-dependent diabetes). But obesity can also predispose men to colon (also known as colorectal) cancer and prostate cancer, and women to endometrial, gallbladder, cervical, ovarian, and breast cancer. As far as specific GI disorders go, obesity can trigger gastroesophageal reflux disease, gallbladder disease, and a range of other problems you'll read about in this book. But many lean and fit people also suffer from chronic GI problems . . . especially if they smoke.

Food allergies and food poisoning are also major sources of GI upset. As our food supply grows more "technological," we're seeing an increasing number of food sensitivities and an increase in food-borne infections. But the most recent infectious disease news has to do with one of the most common GI disorders: stomach ulcers. Long thought to be related to stress, stomach ulcers have now been shown to be caused by the bacteria *Helicobacter pylori* (*H. pylori*).

This book is designed as a life companion. Most of you will be buying it because you currently have a particular symptom or disease. But much of the information in these pages is timeless.

Chapter 1, "How Readers Digest," discusses exactly that: how your digestive system works. Chapter 2, "When You Have That Gut Feeling," will help you sort out whether your symptoms point to an upper or lower GI problem (it's not always obvious). More important, chapter 2 will help you report your symptoms accurately to your doctor and discuss appropriate diagnostic tests. For example, upper GI symptoms can mimic cardiovascular symptoms. Chapter 3 should be read by anyone who thinks she or he has an ulcer, who has been recently diagnosed with an ulcer, or has been diagnosed with an ulcer in the past ten years. Ulcers can recur unless the underlying bacterial infection is treated. I'll also tell you some things I bet you didn't know about taking antibiotics.

Chapter 4, "When the Issue Is NUD and GERD" (as in non-ulcer dyspepsia and gastroesophageal reflux disease), should be read by anyone who has experienced heartburn or abdominal pain that is not linked to an ulcer. This chapter will explain the many causes of heartburn as well as the treatments. Ever taken an antacid or an acid-controlling drug? Or a drug that irritates your stomach? Then let me tell you "About Those Stomach Medicines" in chapter 5.

Moving on down, chapter 6, "Bowels of the Earth," is written for anyone who experiences irregular bowel movements or bowel habits, as well as for those who have been diagnosed with irritable bowel syndrome (IBS) or an inflammatory bowel disease (IBD), such as ulcerative colitis or Crohn's disease. This chapter will help you obtain the right diagnosis or help to explain what's going on if you've been living with these disorders for some time. The latest treatments are discussed, including the use of nicotine patches for controlling ulcerative colitis symptoms. Chapter 6 also discusses who should be screened for colon cancer and some signs to watch for.

Chapter 7, "The Trouble with Abs," covers all of those disorders that are "in between" by virtue of biological geography. Whether you're curious about cirrhosis of the liver, have a hiatal hernia or gallbladder disease, or are worried about appendicitis, this is the chapter to read. Chapter 8, "People in Special Circumstances," addresses other diseases that, while not considered GI disorders per se, cause a host of GI problems. This chapter devotes significant space to eating disorders, people living with HIV/AIDS, as well as female reproductive problems, ranging from endometriosis to symptoms of ovarian cancer—symptoms that are GI in nature.

Chapter 9, "Living Well, Eating Well, Feeling Well" discusses a range of wellness issues from understanding fat and fiber (increase the latter, decrease the fat), phytochemicals, and how to reduce the odds of developing colon cancer and other cancers through diet. The last chapter, "Cancer in the GI Tract" serves as a general introduction to understanding cancer and discusses the kinds of gastrointestinal cancers that can develop, and treatment options.

This book also includes a glossary of terms and a comprehensive resource list with Internet instructions to help you find out more. And as you read through this edition, I'll be busy researching GI news for future editions. In the meantime, feel free to contact me care of my publisher if you need more information. I have lots of other material I'm happy to share with you.

CHAPTER 1

HOW READERS DIGEST

It's difficult to understand the range of gastrointestinal ailments that can affect us if we don't understand how the digestive tract works. In fact, it's amazing that anyone feels well after eating, considering how complicated the act of digesting food really is. The term *digesting* refers to the process by which food is converted into the nutrients we need to live and the excess waste we don't need. Nutrients are the by-product created when food and drink are broken down into their smallest parts to provide energy to our cells.

The digestive tract is a long tube that twists and turns from the mouth to the anus. It is made up of two layers of muscle lined by cells and glands. The cells and glands digest and absorb the nutrients and water from food; the muscles coordinate movement along the system. Two other organs needed for digestion are beside but not part of this tract: the liver and the pancreas. Both these organs are responsible for key digestive juices that reach the small intestine through small connecting tubes.

Essentially, the entire digestive tract (aka gut) is made up of a series of muscles that are triggered at different stages of digestion. The job of these muscles is to coordinate how and when food is moved along the tract. However, many outside factors can interfere with the muscle coordination of the digestive tract. And when that happens, you may not feel well. In fact, more people are hospitalized for gastrointestinal disorders than any other type of disorder.

AN UNREMARKABLE MEAL

The food you eat is not in a usable form for your body. Anything you eat or drink has to be broken down into smaller molecules, nutrients that can be absorbed into the blood and carried to cells throughout the body.

Imagine that your digestive tract is one long subway tunnel with different stops. If you were to look at the GI "subway map," the first stop is your mouth. The next stop is your pharynx, and the third stop is your esophagus. The stomach is a major "connecting stop." This is where the train stops for a while before switching tracks and moving on to the more active parts of your gut: the duodenum, which connects to your small intestine, which connects to the last stop on the line, your large intestine. (See Figure 1.1.)

Chewing Food

The act of chewing actually begins as soon as you smell food. Your salivary glands will begin to secrete saliva, making your mouth water. When you actually taste the food, the saliva really begins to flow. Chewing the food will allow the saliva to mix well with an enzyme called ptyalin, produced by the salivary glands. Ptyalin starts the process of carbohydrate digestion, and the conversion to glucose occurs at the lining of the small intestine. Carbohydrates not digested generally reach the colon, where they ferment. Chewing your food well will help you digest carbohydrates more efficiently.

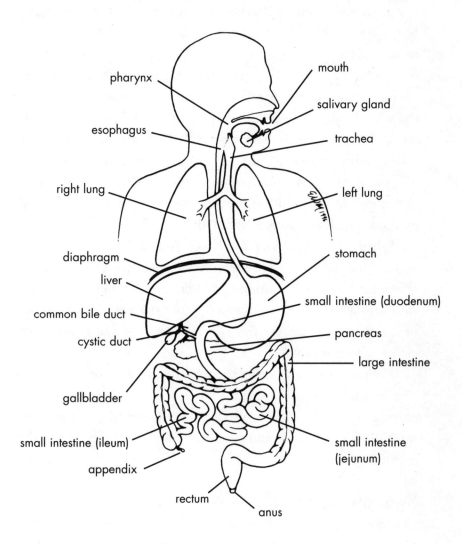

FIGURE 1.1 **The Gastrointestinal Tract**

Illustration by Elizabeth Weadon Massari © 1996.

The more you chew, the more saliva you make. You have three pairs of salivary glands: the parotid glands are under the earlobes, the submaxillary glands are along the side of the lower jawbone, while the submental glands are at the bottom of the mouth. Each of the salivary glands is triggered by the taste of food, which is sensed by taste buds on the tongue. Your molars stimulate the parotid glands to produce the most potent saliva, the saliva containing ptyalin. Salty or bitter foods will also stimulate the parotid glands. The submaxillary glands are triggered by sour or oily/fatty foods, and are also necessary for chewing meat. The submental glands are triggered by sweet foods as well as natural sugars in fruits and vegetables. A thinner saliva is produced by the submental glands to dilute the sweetness.

When you chew your food well (we're supposed to chew about thirty-two times per bite!), you should detect three distinct tastes, known as the beginning, middle, and end tastes. Chewing stimulates your digestive tract to produce digestive juices; the act of chewing also relaxes your nervous system—one reason why eating is so enjoyable.

Chewing well also helps to strengthen the teeth and gums. The parotid glands excrete the hormone parotin, which helps maintain the teeth. Parotin also has other functions, such as stimulating cell metabolism and even increasing T-cell function in the immune system.

Swallowing Food

Swallowing food triggers all the muscles in the digestive tract to begin contracting in wavelike motions known as peristalsis. The act of swallowing is voluntary, but once the food is down the throat, the rest of the movement through the digestive tract is involuntary, or beyond our control. Our nervous system takes over. The food goes down the throat into the pharynx and into the esophagus. The esophagus connects the throat to the stomach.

In order for food to get from the esophagus to the stomach, it must go through a crucial tunnel known as the lower esophageal (pronounced *eso-FA-jeel*) sphincter (LES). The lower esophageal sphincter acts as a valve to prevent stomach contents from regurgitating back into the esophagus. This sphincter opens and shuts through a series of contractions known as *peristalsis*, similar to the contractions that occur when you have a bowel movement. There are two peristaltic waves—primary and secondary—which occur in the esophagus. The LES has to be coordinated so that it relaxes when food passes down and then closes at other times.

The LES opens to allow food to pass. It remains closed at all other times and thus prevents reflux, or "back up." When the LES doesn't work properly, you'll suffer from symptoms of gastroesophageal reflux disease (GERD), which include heartburn, pain, and regurgitation (the feeling of food coming back up).

Digesting Food

The stomach is an accordionlike bag of muscle and other tissue near the center of the abdomen just below the rib cage. The bag expands to accommodate food and shrinks when it is empty. The stomach itself is a "holding tank" for food until it can be distributed into more distant parts of the gastrointestinal tract.

To appreciate what the stomach does, imagine what happens when you make coffee from the whole bean. First, you grind the bean in a coffee grinder. Your stomach does the same thing with the food particles it gets, combining the chewed food with gastric secretions, forming chyme (pronounced *kime*), a semifluid mixture. In the same way that hot water will turn ground coffee into a beverage, three substances (mucus, hydrochloric acid, and pepsin), turn chyme into an even mushier mixture. Too much hydrochloric acid can irritate the stomach (see chapter 3); stress, worry, and anxiety may contribute to excess production of hydrochloric acid.

In the same way that the larger coffee grounds stay in the filter, the larger solid particles of food go from the stomach into the duodenum for further digesting, while the mushy, nicely "worked over" food remnants from the stomach will quickly pass into the small intestine (aka midgut or small bowel). The small intestine is usually called just that, but technically, it consists of three sections: the duodenum, jejunum, and ileum. For the purposes of this book, I will simply refer to the jejunum and ileum as "the small intestine." This entire process is known as gastric emptying.

GI motility

A more technical term for this phase of digestion is known as motility, since what's really happening is that a series of various tubes along the GI tract are emptying food particles from one into the next. This emptying process is dependent on continuous movement, known as *motility*, which is controlled by nerves, hormones, and muscles. If you're experiencing problems with other parts of your endocrine (hormonal) system, such as a thyroid problem, the entire gastric-emptying process can be slowed down (you'll be constipated and bloated) or speeded up (you'll have diarrhea). Gastric emptying can also be affected by what you're eating and by your stomach's muscle movement.

I refer to motility as the "juices and motion" segment of digestion. This means that digestive juices, combined with the natural contractions and waves of all that tubing, are moving food from point A to point B. However, keep in mind that the mechanisms involved in breaking down liquids, solids, and indigestible solids are all different. That's why treating a gastrointestinal disorder is so complicated; depending on which kind of food is not moving through the system, you will need different life-style modifications, therapies, exercises, or treatments.

The small intestine

By the time food gets into the small intestine, it is mushed up by the digestive secretions of the stomach, pancreas, and biliary tract. This mush stays in the small intestine for a relatively long time. One reason is that all the nutrients the body cannot absorb, along with bacteria and cellular debris from the intestine itself, have to be "tagged" here for elimination. Otherwise, this accumulation of waste will interfere with normal intestinal functioning. All the usable nutrients are absorbed through the intestinal walls. These nutrients include digested molecules of food, water, and minerals from the diet. These absorbed nutrients are carried off into the bloodstream, where they go to other parts of the body for storage or further chemical change. The waste products are sent to the large intestine (aka colon or large bowel), where they sit around for a day or two before they are expelled in the form of stools.

Due South

Everything above the large intestine is considered the upper GI tract. Everything below the small intestine is considered the lower GI tract. From the small intestine, all waste products move into the colon, as mentioned above. This is essentially a large dehydrator; it extracts all liquid from the waste and turns it into the recognizable stool. This is a region that is especially twisty; air frequently gets trapped in here, and we pass gas. The stool gets moved along into the rectum, which serves as a holding tank for the stool until we are ready to make the time to sit down, relax, and let it all come out the anus. The anus, like the lower esophagus, has a muscular sphincter, known as the external anal sphincter. Unlike the esophageal sphincter, this is a voluntary sphincter that we can control (thank goodness)! The internal anal sphincter is involuntary and controls continence most of the time when we are not thinking about it.

The colorectum

The large intestine is also known as the colorectum, made up mostly of muscle tissue, but also containing some fat and lymph tissue. This lining is coated by a layer of cells known as the epithelium or mucosa. The epithelium enables the large intestine to absorb liquid from the waste products, and also produces mucus that allows stools to pass. People with bowel disorders may notice that there is mucus in their stools, which may be a sign that the epithelium is overproducing mucus for some reason. If you suddenly notice mucus in your stools, have it investigated to rule out a serious problem.

HAVING A BREAKDOWN

A variety of digestive juices, enzymes, and hormones are responsible for breaking down particular kinds of foods. In general, digestive juices begin in the mouth with saliva, and continue through the stomach lining and small intestine. The pancreas is the chief manufacturer of digestive enzymes needed to break down the carbohydrates, fat, and protein in our food. Other enzymes come from glands in the lining of the intestine. Only a tiny portion of the pancreas makes insulin, a hormone that distributes glucose into the cells of the body. (People who do not make insulin will develop diabetes—but that's another book!)

The liver produces bile, which is stored between meals in the gallbladder (discussed more in chapter 7). Squeezed out of the gallbladder into the bile ducts when you eat, bile is used to break down fat into the watery contents of the intestine (similar to what happens when you use dishwashing liquid to dissolve grease from the broiler). Digestive enzymes from the pancreas mix with bile in the small intestine.

The digestive hormones gastrin, secretin, and cholecystokinin (CCK) control the secretions and function of the digestive system and are released by cells that line the stomach and small intestine. These hormones are released into the bloodstream, head to the heart through the arteries, and wind up back in the digestive system.

Gastrin is what signals the stomach to produce acid, necessary for breaking down food. Gastrin also controls the normal growth of cells and tissue in the stomach lining, small intestine, and colon. Secretin is the hormone that "kick-starts" all the pancreatic juices, which contain bicarbonate. Secretin also signals the stomach to produce pepsin (which breaks down protein) and the liver to produce bile (which breaks down fat). CCK stimulates the pancreas to make enzymes and also causes the gallbladder to empty its bile.

What Nerve

Finally, two sets of nerves control the movement of all these digestive parts, known as the extrinsic (outside) nerves and the intrinsic (inside) nerves. The nervous system is the brains of the digestive system. Extrinsic nerves are from the unconscious part of the brain or the spinal cord. These nerves make the chemicals acetylcholine and adrenaline. Acetylcholine is what makes the digestive tract muscles squeeze the food through all that tubing, while forcing the stomach and pancreas to squeeze out their juices. Adrenaline, on the other hand, smooths out the digestive tract muscles, creating the wavelike movements together with acetylcholine. Adrenaline also decreases blood flow to the stomach and intestine.

Intrinsic nerves are like a network of wires in the linings of the esophagus, stomach, small intestine, and colon. Every time food stretches out these organs, these nerves release a variety of substances that either speed up or delay the movement of food through the digestive tract. If your foods were the "pinball," intrinsic nerves would be the "bumpers."

How You Are What You Eat

The digestive juices you secrete may change depending on what you're eating. Here's a brief overview.

Carbohydrates

Most people in the Western world eat roughly half a pound of carbohydrates per day. Carbohydrates contain both starch and fiber. The fiber is not digestible and is sent to the colon as waste.

The starches in carbohydrates are broken down into simpler molecules by specific enzymes in saliva (ptyalin), the pancreas (amylase), and the lining of the small intestine. Starch is first converted into maltose by maltase, then further split into glucose molecules, which are absorbed into the bloodstream as long as you are making enough insulin and your cells are responding to insulin. Glucose is carried through the bloodstream into the liver, where it is stored or used for energy.

Table sugar (sucrose) is immediately digested into glucose and fructose, both of which are absorbed from the small intestine into the bloodstream.

Milk contains the sugar lactose, which cannot be broken down into an absorbable product without the enzyme lactase.

Protein

Meat, eggs, and beans, all the basic proteins we eat, contain giant molecules that have to be broken down by pancreatic enzymes (protease) into amino acids, smaller molecules the body can absorb.

Fats

Digesting fat involves turning it into a watery substance. Bile, secreted by the liver, which is stored in the gallbladder, is used to help absorb cholesterol but is not a product of fat breakdown. As discussed earlier, bile acts like dishwashing liquid to dissolve fat in water, allowing the fat enzymes to break the large fat molecules into smaller molecules called fatty acids and glycerol or monoglycerides. The bile acids combine with the fatty acids and cholesterol, which move into the cells of the intestinal lining. Here, the small fat molecules are turned back into large molecules, which pass into the lymphatic system. Reconstituted fat goes into the veins of the chest, while the bloodstream carries the other fat into special storage areas throughout the body.

Vitamins

Vitamins are chemicals in food that are classified by the fluids in which they are broken down. Vitamins B and C are considered water-soluble vitamins, because they are dissolved in water, while vitamins A, D, E, and K are fat-soluble vitamins. If you consume too many water-soluble vitamins, they will simply be excreted; too many fat-soluble vitamins will accumulate in the body's tissues.

Water and Salt

All the water and salt you eat is dissolved in the small intestine. Every twenty-four hours, a typical person will absorb more than a gallon of water containing more than an ounce of salt from the intestine.

WHEN THE BREAKDOWN BREAKS DOWN

A range of things can go wrong throughout this complex food breakdown process. If even one hormone or enzyme is "off" in your system, there will be consequences. GI disorders are, themselves, broken down into upper GI disorders and lower GI disorders. Upper GI disorders can include the following.

- **Dysmotility:** Impaired movement of some of the muscles in the GI tract. This can lead to a condition known as gastroesophageal reflux disease (GERD) or hypomotility, where the sphincter at the bottom of the esophagus does not contract enough and lets stomach acid come back up. GERD has a number of causes, ranging from unknown (also called idiopathic) to the overuse of certain drugs. When your GI tract is overactive or hypermotile, you will experience spastic motor disorders because your contractions will be much too strong. This will cause stomach pains and obstructions throughout your GI tract. Therefore, treatment for GERD and hypermotility are opposite. Most people suffer from GERD rather than hypermotility. See chapter 4 for more details.
- **Excess acid:** Too much hydrochloric acid in the stomach may cause an ulcer or hiatus hernia. See chapter 3 for more details on ulcers and chapter 7 for more information on hiatus hernia.
- **Reflux:** This is a fancy word for heartburn and is usually a symptom of either GERD or an ulcer, but reflux could be caused by a perfectly normal occurrence such as pregnancy, for example. This is when semi-digested food comes back up the esophageal sphincter, leaving a bitter taste in the mouth and a burning feeling in the esophagus.

- **Cancer:** Every part of your body is vulnerable to cancer; your digestive tract is no different. While esophageal and stomach cancer are more common than pancreatic cancer, they are still not as common as colon cancer. Symptoms of GI cancers are discussed in the next chapter, but please read far more thorough cancer books if you suspect you are suffering from a GI cancer.

Lower GI Disorders

Many problems can occur once your food gets south of the lower intestine, ranging from minor yet temporary ailments such as gas, diarrhea, or constipation, to serious chronic ailments such as:

- **Inflammatory bowel diseases (IBD):** This includes ulcerative colitis (inflammation of the colon), ileitis, or inflammation of the ileum, or regional enteritis (Crohn's disease), which is technically above the large intestine. Symptoms are discussed in chapter 6.
- **Irritable bowel syndrome:** Far more common in women than in men, this is often a response to stress, which can cause either diarrhea or constipation, or a combination of both. This is not a psychosomatic condition but, rather, triggered by stressful situations. The stress is real and so are the digestive symptoms.
- **Diverticulosis or diverticulitis:** This problem occurs when small pouches on the wall of the colon become inflamed, causing pain and cramping.

For details on all of these and other lower bowel disorders, see chapter 6.

Stress and Digestion

Stress is a major factor that affects your digestion. The golden rule is not to eat when you are in a state of emotional upset. If you must eat during this time, eat foods that are easy to digest, such as fruits and vegetables. Stress can cause your GI tract to oversecrete acid and undersecrete digestive enzymes. Stress can also decrease the peristaltic wave action of the digestive muscles. That's why stomach problems are common in high-stress workplaces or in high-stress situations.

Stress can also affect bowel habits. People also respond to stress with feelings of bloatedness, nausea, and vomiting. University students classically complain of upper GI problems around exam time.

The general Western life-style of too much fat, not enough fiber, and no exercise puts a different kind of stress on the digestive system. This can lead to chronic upper GI problems, such as GERD, Type II diabetes (a disorder in which cells stop responding to insulin, the hormone that gets glucose into the cells), and a variety of GI cancers, such as colon cancer. Chapter 9 provides a number of suggestions for improving your diet and life-style, which in turn will greatly improve your digestive system.

Smoking

Smoking is the shortest route to an upset stomach. Not only does smoking contribute to heartburn and ulcers, but it seems to decrease the pressure of the lower esophageal sphincter, causing GERD and reflux.

Studies show that duodenal ulcers are less likely to heal and more likely to cause death in smokers than in nonsmokers. Most of the stomach acid is neutralized by sodium bicarbonate, an alkaline substance in the duodenum, made by the pancreas. Studies suggest that smoking reduces the bicarbonate produced by the pancreas, so that the acid in the duodenum is not completely neutralized. Studies also show that smoking may increase the amount of acid secreted by the stomach in the first place.

Things That Get in the Way

Your digestive tract shares close space with a range of neighbors. The pancreas, appendix, and liver can all become inflamed, as in (respectively): pancreatitis, appendicitis, and hepatitis (inflammation of the liver due to infection with hepatitis A, B, or C) or cirrhosis (inflammation of the liver due to viral infections, alcohol abuse, or toxins). The gallbladder has a bad habit of "petrifying" the bile it stores into little stones. This results in gallstones or gallbladder disease; it's not fun.

All these conditions will interfere with digestion, causing cramping and pain. You can live a happy and peaceful life without your appendix or gallbladder, so these can be surgically removed. You need your pancreas and liver, however. See chapter 7 for everything you need to know about the symptoms and treatments for each of these problems.

Ladies only

Women have some other things that can get in the way of digestion: their reproductive tract. Many reproductive disorders, such as endometriosis, dysmenorrhea (painful periods), pelvic inflammatory disease, and ectopic pregnancy, will interfere with the digestive tract and may cause a variety of vague cramping and symptoms. Most dangerous are the symptoms of ovarian cancer, characterized by persistent nausea, constipation, and other impossible-to-pin-down signs.

Many normal reproductive functions, ranging from menstruation to pregnancy, can also cause a range of digestive problems. Pregnancy is notorious for heartburn, GERD, and constipation. For more information on gynecological problems, see chapter 8 or consult my book, *The Gynecological Sourcebook*. If you're pregnant and are suffering from GI problems, consult *The Pregnancy Sourcebook*.

Intestinal parasites and bad food

Intestinal parasites or food poisoning can wreak havoc on the digestive system, often causing near-death symptoms. See chapter 8 for more details on sudden and severe gastrointestinal symptoms and how to get emergency attention.

Other diseases and medications

Any serious disease will affect the digestive system, particularly diabetes and AIDS. Thyroid diseases can also affect the digestive tract, and many medications can interfere with the digestive system. The most common side effect of most prescription drugs are "GI in nature"—a common phrase that means diarrhea, constipation, or bleeding from the GI tract. See chapter 8 for more information.

Most of us have experienced a range of minor gastrointestinal upsets along the way. The next chapter is devoted to chronic symptoms that can point to a range of GI disorders, from ulcers and GERD to cancer or other problems in the abdominal region. The next chapter will tell you what you need to know to get diagnosed and treated as quickly as possible without being dismissed with the familiar "It's just stress," or "Eat more fiber"—even though you may be under stress and do need more fiber!

CHAPTER 2

WHEN YOU HAVE THAT GUT FEELING

This chapter is not about having a stomachache. It's about suffering from chronic symptoms in the gastrointestinal tract. "Chronic" refers to symptoms experienced on a regular basis. This can mean a few times a day, a few times a week, or a few times a month. But if you've experienced the symptoms discussed in this chapter only once in your life, or once a year, you do *not* suffer from chronic gastrointestinal symptoms. Chronic GI symptoms can be painful and interfere with daily activities. This is no laughing matter, even though some people treat "heartburn" and "gas" like a joke.

This chapter discusses the most common GI complaints and some of the possible causes behind a variety of symptoms. It also provides you with appropriate questions to ask your doctor, appropriate questions your doctor should be asking *you*, as well as the appropriate diagnostic workup given your symptoms. Finally, this chapter discusses how to get relief and where to go if you need a more thorough investigation.

WHEN YOU'RE BURNING AND BITTER

As discussed in the last chapter, food must pass from the esophagus into the stomach through a sphincter known as the lower esophageal sphincter (LES). For a number of reasons, the sphincter may not completely shut after dumping ingested food particles into the stomach. So what happens? The food, now bathed in stomach acid, can actually come back up through the sphincter, causing a burning sensation in the chest, and even a spreading pain throughout the neck and arms; this pain may be mistaken for a heart attack. You can also experience nausea, belching, and regurgitation of that half-digested food. When it comes back up through the sphincter, it doesn't taste as good as it did going down. Thanks to the acid and enzymes it's been exposed to, the food will taste sour and bitter in your throat. The problem will be aggravated when you bend forward or lie down. In fact, you may find that after an experience like this, you wake up with a sore throat. This problem is clinically called acid reflux, and in lay terms is known as heartburn or acid indigestion.

Heartburn usually lasts about two hours. Most people find that standing up relieves the burning; that's because gravity helps. You could also take an antacid to clear acid out of the esophagus. Not everyone will experience the same degree of heartburn. Heartburn can be mild, moderate, or severe. It all depends on why it's occurring, how often it occurs, when it occurs, and how much food backup you have.

More than 61 million American adults experience heartburn about once a month, while another 25 million suffer from heartburn every day.

Unusual Symptoms

A number of atypical symptoms, which you may not immediately recognize, may suggest that you have reflux. These include morning hoarseness, drooling and coughing spells, as well as waking up with a sore throat. If you have asthma and you find that it suddenly worsens, this could also point to reflux. You could also suddenly have symptoms of asthma when you never suffered from asthma before. In these cases, you may be having reflux at night, which is obstructing your breathing passages, causing all these strange symptoms.

What Causes Heartburn?

There are several causes of heartburn. Sometimes a change in diet will make heartburn disappear. Classic triggers are caffeine, coffee, chocolate, and peppermint, as well as spicy and fatty foods. Citrus and other acidic foods, including tomatoes and juices, can also trigger an episode of heartburn. It's believed that caffeine and peppermint, in particular, can cause the lower esophageal sphincter (LES) to relax, allowing the stomach contents to back up.

We also know that smoking can relax the LES and cause chronic heartburn. In this case, heartburn symptoms won't go away unless you quit smoking or take medication to restore LES motility.

Sometimes heartburn is a symptom of an underlying problem, such as GERD (gastroesophageal reflux disease), discussed more in chapter 4. If this is the case, other symptoms (see further on) may be associated with heartburn, but not always. If heartburn is severe enough to interfere with your daily activities, you will definitely need to alter your life-style significantly to correct the problem or take prescription drugs to reduce acid and/or restore your GI tract's motility.

A perfectly "natural" cause of heartburn is pregnancy. At least 25 percent of all pregnant women suffer from heartburn daily, while half of all pregnant women experience heartburn at some point during their pregnancy. Progesterone relaxes muscular contractions, so that the LES doesn't quite close. Later in pregnancy, as the uterus expands, it pushes the stomach up against the esophagus, thus interfering with the LES's proper functioning.

For the same reasons that pregnancy causes heartburn, so does too much weight in the abdominal region. Again, things get "squished" in what is already a tight area. Too much weight may push up the stomach and cause the LES to relax.

In infancy, formula feeding can be a cause of heartburn, vomiting, coughing, and failure to thrive. Breast-feeding is the remedy; formula-fed babies are much more prone to gastrointestinal upsets such as heartburn than are breast-fed babies.

How Do You Spell R-E-L-I-E-F?

Now might be a good time to read chapter 9. Relieving heartburn is often a question of eating right, quitting smoking, and exercising. Avoiding the "trigger" foods, such as coffee, carbonated drinks, fried and fatty foods, chocolate, alcohol, and peppermint can do wonders. These foods can not only relax the LES, but can irritate the esophageal lining. Gravity helps, too. Elevating the head of your bed about six inches and avoiding lying down after eating can also work well. For temporary relief, you can also take an over-the-counter antacid.

All those television commercials that air around the dinner hour, encouraging you to "have the chili, have the cheesecake," and then take the brand-name antacid, do a great disservice. It's not okay to continue to eat the wrong foods and then take an antacid as a "chaser." As I'll discuss in chapter 5, even the manufacturers of these antacids encourage temporary use and recommend consulting a doctor if symptoms persist. If you're suffering from heartburn because of certain foods, your body is saying: "Hey—quit eating this stuff!"

WHEN YOU HAVE PAIN

Pain in the stomach area (that is, north of the bowel) can point to a variety of problems. What you need to sort out is whether your pain is related to food and whether you find relief with over-the-counter antacids. If your symptoms are more than just heartburn or more localized discomfort, you may be producing far too much acid in your stomach. In this case, you may require a much stronger drug, called an H2 (histamine type 2) receptor antagonist. There's no name for this type of problem other than non-ulcer dyspepsia (NUD). This means discomfort not related to an ulcer. NUD is discussed more in chapter 4.

Pain in the upper GI tract could also mean that you do have an ulcer; this is called peptic ulcer disease (PUD). In this case, you will have a very specific localized area of pain instead of a more generalized feeling of discomfort. Ulcer pain is often relieved by taking antacids and eating small amounts of food, and is aggravated by overeating. Ulcer pain may also wake you up at night; the pain is often described as a gnawing hunger pang that seems to be relieved by milk, ice cream, and other creamy foods.

If you have pain in your stomach region that is more spread out or diffuse, and it gets worse after eating only a small amount of food, then you don't have an ulcer but you may have what's known as dysmotility, a characteristic of GERD, discussed in chapter 4. Motility disorders tend to be diagnosed based on three other symptoms that accompany pain: bloating or abdominal distension, feeling full after eating only a small amount of food, and nausea. Sometimes heartburn will also be present.

The biggest problem is distinguishing ulcer pain from non-ulcer pain. In fact, the symptoms that many doctors classify as typical ulcer pain—such as pain brought on by not eating and relieved by eating, as well as gnawing, burning pain—can also mean you have non-ulcer dyspepsia, especially if classic heartburn seems to accompany the pain. Most doctors will be able to sort out the diagnosis by asking the right questions, or sending you for a test that can rule out or confirm an ulcer. Your doctor will probably try to classify your GI discomfort as ulcerlike, refluxlike, or dysmotilitylike.

What Causes These Pains?

Chapter 3 discusses in detail the causes and treatments for peptic ulcer disease. Stress is now considered to play only a minor role in triggering an ulcer. The causes are indeed physiological, not just rooted in emotions. Classic triggers of ulcerlike pains—that is, when it feels like an ulcer but is not an ulcer—are certain drugs: aspirin or nonsteroidal anti-inflammatory drugs (NSAIDs), such as ibuprofen or acetaminophen. These drugs can also trigger an ulcer, as you'll see in the next chapter.

Non-ulcer pain is often a symptom of a larger underlying condition, such as GERD (see chapter 4), dysmotility (see chapter 4), or just plain bad habits, such as a high-fat diet, lack of exercise, and smoking.

A Number of Symptoms

The most difficult people to diagnose are those with several symptoms. As discussed above, heartburn pain is often accompanied by bloating, feeling full after only a few bites (known as early satiety), nausea, and vomiting. Generally, when these symptoms occur together in this particular bundle, you probably have a motility disorder, meaning that the muscles in your esophagus and stomach region are not coordinating well enough to move food from point A to point B. Motility disorders are usually part and parcel of GERD, which is discussed in chapter 4.

The problem is that many people report only one or two symptoms, such as pain or heartburn, and do not include the other key symptoms: bloating/gas, early satiety, and nausea/vomiting. Some specialists feel that a number of people diagnosed with motility problems actually have irritable bowel syndrome "above the bowel." The patient with upper GI problems may also have lower GI problems. In other words, it's entirely possible to be suffering from GERD as well as irritable bowel syndrome. That's why giving your doctor specific information will help him or her sort out what's really going on.

WHEN YOU HAVE CRAMPS

There is a difference between a pain and a cramp. A cramp comes in bursts and spasms, while a pain is persistent. Gastrointestinal cramps mean that something is not going well in the intestines and will usually be relieved by a bowel movement or a bout of diarrhea. The cramp, in this case, could be caused by gas, or often by bad food: undercooked chicken, old leftovers, or drinking water in places where you're warned, "Don't drink the water." These episodes will usually come and go. If you experience fever and/or vomiting with cramps, it's best to go to an emergency ward to be evaluated for food poisoning. These symptoms can also mean that you have a flu virus.

Suffering from chronic cramping after a meal is often caused by irritable bowel syndrome (IBS). Inflammatory bowel diseases

(IBD) are other common reasons for cramping. In IBD (*not* IBS) bloody diarrhea or stools, as well as fever, chills, weight loss, and nausea accompany the cramps. These miserable conditions are detailed in chapter 6. It's also worth noting that food intolerances can play a role in cramping after eating, a common IBS-related problem; however, this is not the same as an allergy.

Lactose Intolerance

Over 50 million North Americans suffer from an intolerance to milk, known as lactose intolerance. This means that they lack the enzyme lactase, which breaks down the sugar lactose into glucose. Lactose intolerance is extremely common among people of African, Asian, Aboriginal, Mexican, and Jewish descent. With this condition, people will experience cramping, gas, bloating, and diarrhea anywhere from fifteen minutes to three hours after eating any dairy product. The treatment is simple: Avoid eating dairy products. We don't really need to eat dairy products; we can get all the protein and calcium we need from a variety of other foods, discussed in chapter 9. If you want to continue to eat dairy foods, however, simply take Lactaid with your dairy food. This contains the enzyme lactase, which will enable you to digest dairy foods.

Celiac Disease

Celiac disease is a much rarer, inherited disorder, where the body has an inflammatory response in the bowel wall due to the presence of gluten. The bowel is then damaged from the inflammation and this leads to the symptoms below. Gluten is found in wheat, rye, barley, and oats but is not a starch. Potatoes and rice, for example, do not contain gluten. When someone with celiac disease eats gluten, the intestines can be damaged. Symptoms include severe cramping and a pale or watery stool that often floats in the toilet, because the stool contains excess fat that was never absorbed by the body. Celiac disease is also accompanied by bloating, vomiting, muscle wasting, skin rashes, anemia, and lack of appetite. Early satiety (feeling full after only a few bites of food) is another symptom of celiac disease. This is a "masquerader" disease. In fact, people with undiagnosed celiac can be misdiagnosed with any of the following:

- GERD (see chapter 4)
- lactose intolerance (see above)
- ulcerative colitis (see chapter 6)
- Crohn's disease (see chapter 6)
- HIV-related diseases (see chapter 8)

There is a blood test for celiac disease, but it is not widely available and isn't perfect. The best way to diagnose celiac disease is through an intestinal biopsy that involves removing a tiny piece of bowel. The blood test helps, but has not yet reached the stage where it can replace this biopsy. But once celiac disease is diagnosed, the treatment is simple: Avoid gluten-containing foods. This will involve seeing a dietitian and planning a high-protein, high-calorie, gluten-free diet. See Table 2.1 for a list of gluten-containing foods as well as gluten-free foods. Occasionally, people with celiac disease may also be diabetic. In this case, you'll need to meal-plan very carefully with your diabetes educator and dietitian to make sure your blood sugar levels are in check.

Other intolerances

There are dozens of food intolerances that can cause cramping and diarrhea. Many other food allergies, however, cause respiratory symptoms. If you find that you experience cramps, gas, or diarrhea after you eat, record what you eat in a diary so that you can begin to isolate the offending food, whether it's dairy or berry.

TABLE 2.1 **Gluten-Containing and Gluten-Free Foods**
The following table is intended for people with celiac disease or people who suspect they may have celiac disease.

Food Group	Gluten Foods	Gluten-Free Foods
Starches	Pastas, packaged rice mixes, cereals, breads, crackers	Breads/crackers made from rice, corn, or potato flour; cereals made from corn or rice (not malt); rice crackers, plain corn and potato chips, rice cakes, cornmeal tortillas, popcorn
Fruits and Vegetables	Creamed vegetables	Fresh and frozen with no added ingredients; fruit canned in fruit juice; dried fruit
Milk	Malted milk, Ovaltine, some nondairy creamers, desserts, flavored coffees	Fluid milk; evaporated milk, milk powder; real cream, such as whipping, cereal cream
Sugars	Candies, chocolate-coated nuts	Pure jelly, honey, jam, brown and white sugar, corn and maple syrup, molasses, pure cocoa powder
Proteins	Prepared meats (e.g., hot dogs); cheese containing oat gum	All fresh or frozen meats, fish, and poultry with no batter or breading or other pre-preparation; canned fish; eggs; aged cheese, ricotta, cottage cheese; dried peas, beans, and lentils; tofu

TABLE 2.1 (CONTINUED)

Food Group	Gluten Foods	Gluten-Free Foods
Fats	Salad dressings	Butter, margarine, vegetable oils, oil and vinegar dressing
Alcohol	Vodka, ale, beer, gin, whiskey	Wine

Source: Adapted from Jacqui Tofflemire, "Celiac Disease." Diabetes Dialogue 44, no. 1 (Spring 1997): 30.

SYMPTOMS THAT MIGHT INDICATE "ALARM"

There are certain "red flag" symptoms that warrant an immediate investigation by a gastrointestinal specialist; these doctors are called gastroenterologists. Alarming symptoms don't necessarily mean that you have a serious condition; they mean that your physician should *rule out* something serious. The word that distinguishes alarming symptoms from chronic symptoms is *sudden*. If you're between forty-five and fifty-five, and you *suddenly* notice the onset of any of the following symptoms, don't wait to see what happens: Get yourself to a doctor's office as soon as possible, where you can be referred for testing or to a gastroenterologist. For symptoms of colorectal cancer, see chapter 6.

Symptoms that indicate a more serious illness, such as cancer, include:

- weight loss (loss of at least five to ten pounds in the last month without trying)
- vomiting (particularly vomiting blood)

- bloody saliva
- black or bloody stools (black stools indicate the presence of blood)
- anemia (could mean that bleeding is occurring from the GI tract)
- persistent abdominal pain (i.e., nothing makes it go away)
- new and unusual symptoms (particularly if you're over forty-five)
- noticing that food or liquid is sticking in your throat (called dysphagia, or difficulty swallowing)
- feeling full after a few bites (if it's accompanied by heartburn, pain, bloating, and nausea, it's likely to be GERD or a motility disorder, but this is an alarming symptom nonetheless)

When You Have Symptoms Despite Treatment

Another alarm sign is when you notice that even though your doctor has prescribed medication for your GI symptoms, you are not getting better. In this case, it could simply be that the wrong diagnosis was made. It could also mean that there is a more serious, underlying disease at work, which you need to have evaluated as soon as possible.

WHAT TO TELL THE DOCTOR

If you ask gastroenterologists what primary care doctors need to do in order to correctly diagnose a GI disorder, they will say: "Take an accurate history." This phrase does not mean that your doctor has to be a whiz at *Jeopardy*; it means your primary care doctor (general practitioner, family doctor, or internist) must ask you the right questions about your medical history and symptoms in order to determine what's really going on. The problem is, many primary care doctors do not do this, which means that you could be sent for unnecessary tests or referrals. To speed things along, it's important that you report your symptoms accurately. And that's not as easy as it sounds.

A Full Report

Before you begin to report your symptoms, remind your doctor about all the other medical problems you have: allergies, asthma, migraines (often accompanied by nausea), and family history. Chronic problems, such as thyroid disease or diabetes, for example, can definitely affect your digestive system. In addition, other prescription drugs, ranging from antidepressants to nonsteroidal anti-inflammatory drugs (NSAIDs), can affect your GI tract. Tell your doctor whether you take aspirin, acetaminophen, or ibuprofen for commonplace headaches or menstrual cramps. People frequently answer "no" when asked if they're taking medication because they don't realize that this question refers to over-the-counter drugs as well as prescription drugs. And, of course, smoking and alcohol can greatly affect your digestive tract, too. Dieting as well as eating disorders will also affect your digestive tract; it's important to reveal all this information.

Tell your doctor what you do for a living. Long commutes and hectic and stressful schedules can be associated with unusual eating habits. If you're eating on the run, skipping breakfast, and hitting the couch after work, these habits may contribute to your symptoms.

A Dozen Good Questions

It's important to ask yourself the following before you report your symptoms to your primary care doctor:

1. Do you notice symptoms before or after you eat?
2. Does food seem to aggravate or relieve your symptoms?

3. What are you eating before you notice symptoms?
4. Are you a coffee drinker?
5. Do you consume alcohol?
6. Do you have other symptoms associated with meals, such as early satiety, nausea, or vomiting?
7. Do your symptoms wake you up at night? (Suggests an ulcer.)
8. Does rest seem to help?
9. Does lying down make your symptoms worse?
10. Do you notice any drool when you wake up? (Suggests GERD at night.)
11. Is your voice hoarse when you wake up or do you wake up with a cough? (Suggests reflux at night.)
12. Do you have a sore throat when you wake up? (Suggests reflux at night.)

What Relieves Your Symptoms?

A key point to stress in reporting your symptoms is what relieves them. For example, if an over-the-counter antacid helps your symptoms, then it's pretty clear that regardless of whether you have an ulcer or not, you have acidlike dyspepsia (discomfort). If creamy foods relieve your symptoms, then you probably have ulcerlike dyspepsia. If gravity seems to help (standing up versus lying down), combined with antacids, than you have dysmotility-like dyspepsia.

If your GI symptoms can be categorized into these three general groupings, then the doctor can begin to treat the symptoms, often without sending you for further testing or referrals.

As discussed earlier, if you've been prescribed medication for your symptoms but you're not getting better, it's crucial to say so. One of the most common problems gastroenterologists see is a person who complained of heartburn to the family doctor, took medication (antacids or an H2 receptor antagonist), but still has symptoms. Often only heartburn was treated, rather than a larger problem, such as GERD or a motility disorder (chapter 4). Often, primary care doctors simply fail to counsel their patients about diet and life-style modifications that can prevent heartburn from returning.

What Your Doctor Should Ask

Your doctor's questions should include all of the dozen questions you ask yourself before the doctor visit. Doctors should also ask you the following:

1. How old are you? (Some symptoms are more alarming if you're older than forty-five.)
2. Have you ever had these symptoms before?
3. What triggers these symptoms (such as certain foods, timing of meals)?
4. Have you noticed a worsening of symptoms or do your symptoms appear to be the same?
5. What does your pain feel like (if you have pain)?
6. Do you notice regurgitation (food coming back up) or nausea after a meal? (Indicates a motility disorder.)
7. Can you finish a normal-size meal without difficulty? (A "no" answer indicates a motility disorder.)
8. Do you notice any bloating after you eat? (Indicates a motility disorder.)
9. Do you notice hunger pangs throughout the day or at night? (Indicates an ulcer.)
10. Do you feel that food is sitting in your stomach and not emptying? (Indicates a motility disorder.)
11. How is your appetite? (Helps distinguish whether you answered question 7 consistently.)

12. Are your symptoms worse or better after eating a small meal? (Helps distinguish ulcer from GERD.)

13. How long have you had these symptoms or noticed them? (Why are you here now versus last week?)

14. How do your symptoms relate to other activities such as work or exercise?

15. What do you do to get relief? (Helps distinguish between ulcer and GERD.)

16. Does belching, passing gas, or having a bowel movement help? (Most people will be embarrassed to say this when answering question 15.)

17. How do you feel when you're standing upright or lifting something? (Is the discomfort posture-related? If so, it's probably not an ulcer.)

18. What type of foods do you normally eat? (Chocolate, peppermint, fatty foods, carbonated drinks can all trigger heartburn.)

19. How often are you going to the bathroom? (Are you constipated?)

20. Have you gained weight in the last year or so? (Abdominal weight is often a trigger for GERD.)

When your doctor says "NSAID"

If your symptoms are related to taking a lot of nonsteroidal anti-inflammatory drugs (NSAIDs), such as ibuprofen or Naprosyn, you may be told to go off the NSAID for a couple of weeks to see if the symptoms subside. If they do, then you know that NSAIDs cause GI upset for you, and you can ask for some other drug as an alternative. Doing an upper GI series (see further on) for someone who has been taking NSAIDs is not very accurate. It's best to reevaluate the symptoms when you're off NSAIDs altogether.

When you're told "it's stress"

It's extremely common to report GI symptoms to your family doctor, or even to go to an emergency room with severe symptoms, only to be sent home with the frustrating diagnosis of "stress." Stress does play a role in GI upset, but it's not a diagnosis. And often, a doctor will clearly state that stress "may be a factor" but you will *hear* "stress is the cause"—when that's not what was said. Regardless of how stress was explained in relation to your GI disorders, the best response is: "Are you going to treat me for acid-dyspepsia, reflux-dyspepsia, or dysmotility?"

Confusing GI symptoms with heart disease

If you've run to your doctor's office or an emergency room complaining of chest pain after walking or some other physical activity, only to find that you have a GI problem, you're not alone. GERD can cause radiating pains throughout the chest, choking spells, and coughing at night—symptoms that could make you think "heart attack." The key question to ask yourself is whether your chest pain is accompanied by:

- shortness of breath
- palpitations
- sweating

If the answers are "no," make sure you report this to your doctor; if any answer is "yes," say so. That could make the difference between undergoing a stress test in a cardiologist's office or cutting down on chocolate and peppermint.

DIAGNOSTIC TESTS

If your doctor can figure out whether your symptoms are related to acid/ulcer, reflux, or dysmotility (which is part and parcel of GERD), there's probably no reason to order any tests unless you have alarming symptoms, as discussed earlier. (See Table 2.2.) Your doctor can go ahead and treat you. But if there is some confusion about what you have, then it's probably a good idea to send you to a gastroenterologist for an evaluation. In turn, this specialist may send you for tests to rule out or confirm various diagnoses. These tests can include:

- **An upper GI series.** This means that the doctor takes a series of images followed by a barium tracer, to get a picture of what's going on in your upper GI tract. This should be the "first stop" in GI testing. The X rays will include the esophagus, stomach, and duodenum. This test will rule out an ulcer, but it won't tell the doctor anything about acid or motility. Your doctor can get some information about how the esophagus contracts, and can tell if there's any decreased activity in elderly patients or in people with diabetes. But unless you have really severe gastric discomfort, where you may have leftover food particles in your stomach, for example, these tests won't tell much about motility.
- **Endoscopy.** Here, a thin, lighted tube is passed down the throat and esophagus. This test is a good idea if you have chronic heartburn because it will tell your doctor whether your heartburn has caused esophagitis (inflammation of the tissue lining the esophagus). If your heartburn is bad enough to cause inflammation, the doctor should "treat aggressively" with a very strong antacid drug, such as an H2 receptor antagonist. In other words, over-the-counter antacids probably aren't strong enough in this case.

TABLE 2.2 **Why All the Tests?**
The following table outlines the symptoms that warrant each test.

Endoscopy

To find esophagitis; to rule out ulcer, other mucosal damage, strictures, organic lesions (including cancer); also used (with biopsy or blood work) to determine malignancy; recommended for relapsers or nonresponders after therapy, patients who develop complications of ulcer or esophagitis, or patients over forty with "red flag" symptoms.

Radiography (barium swallow)

To rule out cancer, ulcer, structural abnormalities; checks for ulcers in the stomach or duodenum; indicated for people with difficulty swallowing who have heartburn.

Esophageal pH monitoring

Most useful for linking atypical symptoms with heartburn in patients who are not responding to treatment.

Acid perfusion (Bernstein test)

To determine esophageal sensitivity to acid; reserved for patients with atypical symptoms.

Esophageal manometry

Useful prior to antireflux surgery to rule out a motor disorder; also useful for patients who have trouble swallowing or have atypical symptoms.

Gastric-emptying testing or gastric manometry

Used to determine a motility disorder, or the site or nature of suspected dysmotility.

Sources: Adapted from CMA Patient Counselling Series. W. G. Paterson, editor, Non-ulcer Upper Gastrointestinal Disorders. Grovenor Press, 1995: 46–47.

▣ **Biopsy.** This shouldn't be necessary unless you have confusing results from endoscopy, coupled by alarming symptoms. In this case, a tiny piece of tissue that lines the esophagus is removed for investigation.

▣ **The Bernstein test.** This is when your doctor wants to "drop acid." Here, a mild acid is dripped through a tube that's placed about midway down your esophagus. This test isn't usually necessary if a good history is done, but the purpose is to confirm whether the symptoms are a result of contact between your esophageal lining and acid.

- **Scintigraphy.** This is a gastric-emptying test that involves nuclear medicine. Here, you eat some eggs that have been scrambled with radioactive technetium. After you swallow the eggs, a gamma counter determines how quickly the eggs empty out of your stomach.
- **Esophageal manometry.** This measures the motility of the esophagus by measuring the pressure within the esophagus. This is best for people with atypical symptoms or those with difficulty swallowing.
- **pH testing.** The acid levels inside your esophagus can be measured through pH testing, a valid test for evaluating GERD or atypical chest pain.

Testing for Motility

There is no useful test to check for a motility disorder. The only way this can be done is by taking a careful history—asking the right questions. In people with motility problems, upper GI series, endoscopy, and even gastric-emptying tests are often normal. If this is what your doctor thinks is going on, then treating the problem with a trial course of therapy using a prokinetic drug (meaning a "pro-movement" drug) such as cisapride is the appropriate way to manage the problem.

WHAT'S THE TREATMENT?

Roughly 40 to 60 percent of all people who have heartburn symptoms seem to do well with modifying their life-style (see chapter 9) and taking over-the-counter antacids as needed. Non-prescription antacids provide temporary relief only, and should not be considered first-line therapies unless you have only occasional symptoms. As discussed in chapter 5, using these antacids for long periods of time (longer than two to three weeks) can cause more problems, including diarrhea, as well as too much calcium or magnesium in your system.

If the problem is more than heartburn, and GERD or a motility disorder is suspected, than an H2 receptor antagonist or cisapride, a prokinetic agent (Propulsid in the United States; Prepulsid in Canada), is often prescribed. Cisapride is discussed more in chapter 4. If heartburn symptoms persist, sometimes a more powerful drug, known as a proton pump inhibitor, such as omeprazole or lansoprazole, is prescribed. Combination therapy (an H2 receptor antagonist and cisapride, for example) may be prescribed.

You may require these drugs for a short course of therapy until you're healed, and then practice some better life-style habits, or you may be on these drugs longer. It all depends on how severe your symptoms were to begin with, as well as your individual doctor's philosophy.

The last resort, which very few people will ever need, is surgery, known as an antireflux operation.

If your doctor tells you that you have GERD or non-ulcer dyspepsia (NUD), then you should turn to chapter 4, which discusses these conditions in more detail. If your doctor thinks that the problem is an ulcer, you will need to be investigated for a bacterial infection known as *Helicobacter pylori*. In addition to treatment for your ulcer pain, you'll also be treated with antibiotics for *H. pylori* infection. This is covered in the next chapter.

CHAPTER 3

"I'VE GOT AN ULCER"

The word *ulcer* means that a small surface of an organ or tissue has sloughed off, resulting in a sore. Dozens of types of ulcers can occur in the human body; only about 20 percent of all ulcers are in the gastrointestinal tract. Here, a small part of the lining of the duodenum (in about 90 percent of the cases), esophagus (about 5 percent of cases, a complication of GERD), or the stomach itself (called a gastric ulcer, from the Greek *gaster*, in 5 percent of cases) has somehow worn away. Barrett's esophagus is a condition where the normal lining of the esophagus is replaced by a lining more like the stomach or intestinal lining. It may or may not have ulcers associated with it. Ulcers in the esophagus (called *ulcerative esophagitis*) is a complication of GERD. It is estimated that one in ten North Americans develops an ulcer at some time. The proportion of gastric to duodenal ulcers is somewhat age-dependent and varies. However, gastric ulcers are more common in older patients. Yet, despite the fact that ulcers are not more common, everybody seems to know something about ulcers. When you finish this chapter, you may not believe how much misinformation you've heard through the GI grapevine.

Most people find it disturbing to discover they are the proud owners of an ulcer. That's because of all the folklore surrounding ulcers, which I discuss further on. The most important piece of news about ulcers is that they can now be cured; as recently as the 1970s and 1980s, ulcers were considered chronic conditions that required the sufferer to eat bland foods and take antacids with milk.

Most of us recall only male relatives with ulcers: our fathers, uncles, or grandfathers; that's because ulcers tend to affect men (age forty-five to sixty-five) about twice as often as women. It was presumed that because men don't express their emotions as freely as women, an ulcer formed from bottled-up emotions and stress. This doesn't sound all that illogical, given that the stomach tends to make more hydrochloric acid when we're upset or under stress. Nevertheless, this explanation has been proved wrong.

Ulcers, ladies and gentlemen, are now believed to be caused by a bacterial infection called *Helicobacter pylori* (*H. pylori*). When the infection is treated with antibiotics, the ulcer will almost always go away forever, but there is a small reinfection rate. As we age, we are more likely to have *H. pylori* in our bodies. In fact, the incidence rate equals one's age. At age twenty-five, you have a 25 percent chance of having *H. pylori*; at age fifty, you have a 50 percent chance of having it. Ulcers affect more men than women for reasons that simply are not known. Experts muse whether estrogen and progesterone somehow protect women from ulcers, but no clear research exists as to why ulcers tend to favor the male body over the female. (There are certainly dozens of other conditions that affect more women than men, which we also can't explain!) Furthermore, there are plenty of women with ulcers, too. In fact, *H. pylori* incidence is equal among men and women, although many people with *H. pylori* never develop an ulcer.

This chapter will explain everything you could ever want to know about peptic ulcer disease (PUD), known in lay terms as simply "ulcers." You'll find out what causes ulcers, how they're treated and, ultimately, cured. You'll also find out who is most at risk for developing an ulcer. As for *H. pylori*, you'll find out when it is—and is not—appropriate to be screened for this bacteria, which is usually pretty harmless, as well as what antibiotics will be used to eradicate it. Finally, since there is a lot of misinformation about antibiotic therapy, I recommend that you read the section "Take Only as Prescribed"; antibiotics won't work unless you do this!

ULCERS 101

If you recall from chapter 1, once food reaches the stomach (assuming it doesn't come back up the esophagus), it's ground up by forceful contractions of the stomach muscles, and then mixed with acid and the enzyme pepsin—hence the term *peptic*. Your stomach lining is built of a tough material that can contain the acid and pepsin, which are substances powerful enough to turn a piece of meat into a milkshake. However, if even a tiny portion of your stomach's lining wears away for some reason, then you'll feel the acid and pepsin in the form of symptoms.

Shapes and Sizes

Think about what happens when you get a blister on your foot from new shoes. The blister itself is very tender, forming a deep cavity. The area around the blister becomes a little red and inflamed, which is why it feels itchy. An ulcer is similar. When something wears down the lining of the duodenum, a "blister" or ulcer crater will form there, often one to two inches wide and surrounded by an inflamed area, the walls or margins of the crater.

As mentioned above, about 90 percent of all ulcers form in the duodenum. Therefore, you may be told that you have a duodenal ulcer instead of a peptic ulcer; but they're the same thing. Esophageal ulcers are usually smaller than duodenal or gastric ulcers.

Symptoms

It's possible to have an ulcer without knowing it because ulcers don't always cause symptoms. If you do have symptoms, it's usually a localized pain in the upper GI tract area. Many people find that this pain resembles a hunger pang that often wakes them up at night. The pain may be partially or completely relieved by eating food or by taking antacids. Ulcer pain is usually worse on an empty stomach. Classic ulcer pain tends to strike late in the morning, late in the afternoon, and about three in the morning. Eating food helps because it buffers the acid (as do antacids).

In general, any stomach pain that is strong enough to wake you up is more likely to be an ulcer, because the GI tract "goes to sleep" at night when you do, and usually only wakes up when you do, too. That's why a morning bowel movement is like the "rooster crow" for so many. If you were to define the severity of the pain on a basis of 1 to 5, you'd probably rate this pain as a 2 or 3.

Less common symptoms

Nausea, vomiting (sometimes vomiting blood; sometimes throwing up a meal you ate two days ago), lack of appetite, and weight loss can accompany ulcer pain. "Red flag" symptoms that require an immediate visit to the doctor are when you notice that your stools are blacker than normal or "tarry" (this indicates that there is blood in the stools), or that they have a foul odor (fouler than usual, that is). Dizziness, weakness or paleness (a sign of anemia), and severe back pain (the pain is traveling) are also serious. Some of the symptoms of ulcers are on the "red flag" list in the previous chapter; that's because once an ulcer has developed, it's important to treat it before it gets worse.

Anyone who was a *thirtysomething* fan (yes, I admit it) may recall the episode devoted to Ellen's ulcer. Ellen (played by Polly

Draper) would get up in the middle of the night (again, ulcer pain tends to wake you up), stagger to her bathroom and guzzle milk of magnesia (probably the sponsor!). Feeling dizzy and weak, she had to grab hold of the sink to avoid falling down. When she threw up bright red blood in the sink, she finally accepted the fact that, yes, something was terribly wrong. She was diagnosed with a "bleeding ulcer"; that is, her ulcer was bad enough to cause GI bleeding, which is why she vomited blood. Then she was referred for psychiatric counseling to deal with her stress. The weakness and dizziness were caused by anemia, usually a sign of internal bleeding. (Women with heavy menstrual flows may also become anemic.) As for the stress counseling, it just goes to show you how dated some of those '80s shows are; *thirtysomething* aired in the "pre-*H. pylori* era," if you will, when stress was believed to be a major cause of ulcers.

What Causes the Lining to Break Down?

Studies show that over 90 percent of all people with duodenal ulcers are infected with *H. pylori*, as are more than 70 percent of all people with gastric ulcers. This is discussed in more detail toward the end of this chapter. The theory is that *H. pylori* weakens the lining of the GI tract, making it easier for acid to "break through" or other agents to wear down the lining. That said, there are millions of people walking around with *H. pylori* who will never develop an ulcer. Why is *H. pylori* more potent in some people than others? No one is sure, but it's likely that *H. pylori*, when combined with another trigger—such as certain irritating medications, smoking, or even a genetic predisposition to ulcers (studies show that ulcers run in families)—will become potent. It's like what happens when you combine two ingredients in baking; alone, neither ingredient could make the cake rise, but when they're combined, the cake rises beautifully. Experts also believe that there are different strains of *H. pylori*—some more "vicero-genic" than others.

H. pylori bacteria are shaped like the letter S and live in the mucus that lines the stomach. The longer you have *H. pylori* living inside you, the more time it has to wear down your lining's resistance to its own acid and pepsin. The resistance of the stomach lining to acid and pepsin is lowered when you regularly take aspirin or other nonsteroidal anti-inflammatory drugs (NSAIDs), ranging from ibuprofen to Naprosyn. If NSAIDs are the reason you have an ulcer, you need to weigh the obvious detriment against any potential benefit.

Alcohol can definitely lower the resistance of the stomach lining to acid and pepsin. That includes the alcohol in various medications. Smoking definitely helps to wear down the stomach lining also. Smokers are 50 percent more likely to develop stomach or duodenal ulcers than are nonsmokers. Ulcers also take longer to heal in smokers.

And sometimes your family can "wear down" your stomach lining. Studies show that if a family member develops a gastric or duodenal ulcer, you're likely to as well. At one point, it was thought that there was a genetic predisposition to having less resistant or "thinner" stomach linings. It's more likely that family members infect one another with *H. pylori*, and that's why ulcers run in families. Similarly, colds and flus will also attack a household.

Age is also a factor in ulcers. Ulcers tend to occur after age forty-five, especially in men. Again, there's no clear reason why ulcers favor men over women, but more men take aspirin as blood thinners than women do, while men also tend to drink more alcohol. Ulcers occurring after age forty-five tend to be related to NSAIDs. That said, ulcers can certainly occur in people younger than forty-five and in children.

What about stress?

The more stress you're under, the more likely you are to take aspirin and ibuprofen because you may find you get stress-related headaches. It's also known that you produce more hydrochloric acid when you're under stress. The problem is, ulcers are not actually caused by excess acid; they're caused by a worn-down lining. In fact, some researchers believe that both too much and too little acid and pepsin can lead to an ulcer.

If you take aspirin, you're more likely to develop a stomach or gastric ulcer than a duodenal ulcer—especially if you take more than four aspirins per week for a period of three months. The flip side is that many people take aspirin as a blood thinner to lower their risk of cardiovascular problems. Again, you need to weigh your ulcer against your risk of cardiovascular disease. (Better yet, why don't you change your diet and cut out the aspirin? See chapter 9.)

Esophageal Ulcers

The causes for ulcers in the esophagus are related to heartburn and reflux. The esophagus was not meant to contain acid at all. Therefore, in persons suffering from heartburn/reflux (see chapter 2) or gastroesophageal reflux disease (see chapters 2 and 4), severe reflux could cause an ulcer in the esophagus. Such ulcers account for only 5 percent of all gastrointestinal ulcers.

ULCER FOLKLORE

Since the discovery of *H. pylori,* we can now put to rest a lot of the old myths surrounding ulcers. Here are some of the more popular ones.

MYTH: Stress causes ulcers.

FACT: People who take a lot of aspirin or nonsteroidal anti-inflammatory drugs are far more likely to develop ulcers. People often take these drugs for headaches, which can be brought on by stress. Smokers are also more likely to develop ulcers, and people tend to smoke more when they are under stress. Finally, people who consume alcohol are more likely to develop ulcers; people drink more when they are under stress.

MYTH: Ulcers are more common in lower-class neighborhoods.

FACT: People in low-income groups smoke more and drink more; factors that can predispose them to ulcers. People in low-income groups often share close quarters, which means that if one neighbor is infected with *H. pylori*, it's more likely that this person will infect others. The rules of "public health" hold true for *H. pylori*, as they do for other infectious diseases.

MYTH: If you have an ulcer, you have to be on a bland diet.

FACT: Not in this decade. When my grandfather (who was a doctor) had an ulcer back in the 1970s, he would insist on only bland food and said that he couldn't tolerate spices. We now know that the only things that absolutely irritate an ulcer are alcohol and coffee. Ulcers are treated with powerful acid-blocking drugs, as well as antibiotics to eradicate *H. pylori* infections. (See further on.) After that, most ulcers disappear. What you eat has nothing to do with an ulcer.

MYTH: Milk will heal an ulcer.

FACT: Milk will certainly help to coat the stomach, which could relieve a bout of ulcer pain. But milk will also produce more acid in the stomach. The fact is, most people find that eating *any* food will help relieve ulcer pain when it's in "flare," not just dairy food.

MYTH: *Stomach ulcers cause cancer.*
FACT: This is not true. What happens is that a malignant tumor in the stomach could be missed because of an ulcer; they often look alike on an X ray. That's why it's standard procedure to order an endoscopy (see chapter 2) about six to eight weeks after a gastric ulcer has healed; duodenal ulcers are *rarely* cancerous.

MYTH: *Gastritis is another word for "ulcer."*
FACT: This is not so; gastritis literally means "inflammation of the stomach lining." The confusion between the terms *gastritis* and *ulcer* has come about because the causes of gastritis and an ulcer are the same: *H. pylori,* as well as NSAIDs, aspirin, and alcohol. The symptoms of gastritis are generally nausea, vomiting, and more of a stomach "ache" rather than sharp pain. By treating *H. pylori* (see further on), gastritis has been shown to disappear.

MYTH: *Ulcers cannot be cured.*
FACT: In the 1970s ulcers were treated with bland diets, which did not help. By the 1980s powerful acid-blocking drugs began to be used to treat ulcers; the ulcers would heal but then would come back. When *H. pylori* was discovered, researchers found that by treating the bacteria as well as using an acid-blocking drug, the ulcer would heal and never return about 90 percent of the time. (That was great news, considering that before *H. pylori,* ulcers recurred 50 to 80 percent of the time within one year.) We also know more about NSAID use and ulcers today, which may account for a lower relapse rate.

WHEN YOUR DOCTOR SUSPECTS AN ULCER

In the previous chapter, I devoted considerable space to how to report GI symptoms to your doctor. I suggested appropriate questions for you to ask your doctor, and appropriate questions your doctor should ask you. All those questions regarding how your symptoms relate to food will help tell your doctor whether an ulcer is likely. Gastroenterologists should follow up on their ulcer "hunch" by screening you for *H. pylori* infection using a simple breath test. (*H. pylori* can also be found with a simple blood test.) If you test positive for *H. pylori*, you'll be treated with antibiotics as well as a proton pump inhibitor, such as omeprazole or lansoprazole (see chapter 5).

When Ulcer Is Not Obvious

Many people will not have obvious ulcer symptoms but may notice symptoms of bloating or inability to finish a meal. This could mean that they have non-ulcer dyspepsia (NUD). It could also mean that there is a motility disorder at work. A doctor who is unsure about what's going on will probably want you to have a GI series (X rays following a barium "chaser") and/or an endoscopy procedure that will enable the doctor to see your stomach lining clearly as well as hunt for signs of a previous ulcer. A small sample of the stomach lining can also be obtained, and it can be screened for *H. pylori* as well. See chapter 2 for more details on diagnostic testing.

Some doctors may decide to narrow down the diagnosis by simply treating you with an H2 receptor antagonist, which should work if in fact you have an ulcer. Then, if you don't get better, your doctor will go to "Plan B," which may be to try a different drug or proceed with another investigation. It depends on the circumstance. While this philosophy sounds somewhat half-baked, when it comes to GI therapy it's actually a good management approach. Diagnostic tests, as discussed in the previous chapter, are useful in ruling out an ulcer or a more serious disease. If you have other symptoms on top of ulcer symptoms, you may have GERD or dysmotility (see chapter 4), conditions that are hard to diagnose based on tests. In short, an H2 receptor drug can beautifully sort out whether or not you have an ulcer, because you'll either get better or you won't.

It's important to note that H2 receptor drugs won't work unless you take them properly. They should be taken at night if you have an ulcer. If you also have symptoms of GERD, it will help to divide the dose over the day, so that you're taking it at least twice a day.

Ulcer plus

It's also possible to have an ulcer and another disorder at the same time. For example, you could have a motility problem as well as an ulcer, especially if you find that you continue to suffer from nausea. In this case, the fact that you're not getting better on the H2 receptor drug, coupled with the continuing symptoms, should tip off your doctor that you have what I've coined "ulcer plus"—an ulcer plus another GI disorder.

In this case, your doctor may put you on combination therapy: an H2 receptor antagonist as well as a prokinetic drug to help get your GI tract moving properly again.

When Ulcers Are Emergencies

Any sign of bleeding is an emergency. The symptoms of bleeding, as discussed earlier, include dizziness, weakness, and paleness (all due to anemia), vomiting of blood, or passing black or foul-smelling stools. You've probably heard the one about ulcers "punching a hole through the stomach." Well, this can happen in rare and severe situations. In this case, the ulcer can "furrow" beyond the lining of the stomach or duodenum, into the actual wall that separates the stomach or duodenum from the rest of the abdominal cavity, causing GI bleeding. If the ulcer goes beyond the stomach wall, the stomach acid and other juices can get into the abdominal cavity, which would be an emergency situation requiring immediate treatment. You'd be in a lot of pain and would probably need surgery to repair the hole or perforation. Sometimes an ulcer that perforates through the wall of the stomach or duodenum is a sign of an ulcerating tumor, not a usual stomach ulcer.

An ulcer can also block important pathways through which food needs to go in order to be digested. This is a pretty rare event, but the symptoms would include vomiting up food eaten days ago, while stomach pain would spread throughout the abdominal cavity. This is another case where surgery may be necessary.

THE NEW INFECTIOUS DISEASE

In the mid-1990s, something happened to the entire management and treatment of ulcers that turned GI medicine upside down: Ulcers were proved to be an infectious disease, caused by the bacteria *Helicobacter pylori*. Not only did *H. pylori* make gastroenterology a suddenly "exciting" specialty, but it shifted the "ulcer paradigm" from a stress-related condition to an infectious condition. In other words, patients with ulcers are no longer sent for stress-counseling; instead, they're sent to a pharmacy for a prescription of two or more antibiotics. Ulcer patients are counseled, though, about NSAIDs, aspirin, smoking, and alcohol. All of these things will aggravate an ulcer, as discussed earlier.

Ulcers are therefore cured by antibiotics, but acid-controlling drugs must also be used to treat the symptoms. In other words, the acid-blocking drug is the "Band-Aid"; the antibiotic is the ointment.

Who Found *H. Pylori*?

H. pylori escaped the attention of medical science because it was believed that the stomach was too hostile an environment for any organism to live in. But thanks to the curiosity of an Australian gastroenterologist by the name of Barry J. Marshall, *H. pylori* was discovered circa 1983. Marshall noticed this S-shaped (or even mop-shaped) bug in the stomach tissue of ulcer patients. He decided that the best study would be to swallow the bug itself and see what happened. Sure enough, he developed an ulcer. Further study found that *H. pylori* lives in the stomach's mucous lining, which provides protection from its digestive juices. But by living in the stomach lining, *H. pylori* helps to cause the lining to break down. The good news is that *H. pylori* does not appear to be a sexually transmitted disease. Researchers think it's passed from person to person. Coughing and sneezing might do it. As for oral sex, no one thinks *H. pylori* lives in the genital area, but there are signs that fecal material could carry *H. pylori*. One bad restaurant experience could pass it along; but then, there are so many other horrible things living in fecal material, you'd be more likely to suffer from more dangerous bacteria before *H. pylori* got to you.

Who Is Infected with *H. Pylori*?

Oh, about half the world! In the United States, that translates into about 40 million people, out of whom 10 to 20 percent will ever develop an ulcer. People who live together or who share close quarters are more vulnerable to *H. pylori* infection, for the same reasons they are susceptible to various flu and cold viruses. People who sneeze, cough, and kiss together may find they have ulcers in common. In fact, it's been a well known fact since the 1950s that family members of ulcer patients are three times more likely to develop an ulcer than are those in the general population.

History even records "ulcer outbreaks" similar to influenza outbreaks in various neighborhoods. A famous outbreak occurred during the London bombings of World War II; at that time, stress was blamed for the outbreak.

Perhaps one of the most important groups found to have *H. pylori* were those with some types of stomach cancer. In fact, *H. pylori* infection may triple the risk of developing certain stomach cancers (usually uncommon) even if no ulcers are present.

When Ulcers Come Back

H. pylori has also changed the way past ulcers are treated. For example, if you had an ulcer ten years ago and have not had a recurrence of symptoms, you should still be screened for *H. pylori* infection and treated. That's because *H. pylori* plus a past history of ulcers equals a new ulcer. In fact, unless *H. pylori* is eradicated, the rate of an ulcer recurrence is 60 to 80 percent in the first year without any other therapy.

Studies also show that a strong acid-controlling drug, known as a proton pump inhibitor, can heal both a peptic ulcer and chronic heartburn within four to eight weeks of therapy, as well as preventing either condition from returning. The most common proton pump inhibitor is omeprazole; lansoprazole was recently released in the United States and Canada. There is also a third drug, pantoprazole, which was just released in Canada but has not yet been released in the United States. In fact, lansoprazole heals duodenal ulcers better than H2 receptor drugs, such as ranitidine or famotidine. And that healing rate occurs even when *H. pylori* infection is present. Yet proton pump inhibitors must be prescribed as "maintenance" in order to work. By taking a short course of antibiotics, you can have your ulcer healed without the need to take any more medication.

Shouldn't Everyone Be Screened for *H. Pylori*?

No; many people will test positive for *H. pylori,* but only a few will ever develop ulcers, and only a fraction will develop stomach cancer. Screening and treating everybody for *H. pylori* infection is not only impractical, but no health care system could possibly afford it. In the United States, imagine how much money it would cost to screen the entire population and treat the 40 million people with *H. pylori* with two or three kinds of antibiotics. We're talking billions and billions of dollars. (See Table 3.1.)

The only people who need to be treated for *H. pylori* infection are those who have ulcers or selected people who have chronic non-ulcer dyspepsia; new recommendations found that this group seemed to benefit from *H. pylori* treatment, too. But for the most part, people with other GI disorders, ranging from GERD to appendicitis, don't need to even think about *H. pylori*. It's generally just an "ulcer thing."

Researchers believe that there are different strains of *H. pylori* as well as secondary factors that, when combined with the bacteria,

TABLE 3.1 **Who Should Be Treated for *H. Pylori*?**

If You Have	And are *H. pylori* positive, should you receive treatment?
No ulcer	No
Non-ulcer dyspepsia	Sometimes
Gastric ulcer	Yes
Duodenal ulcer	Yes

trigger an ulcer. For example, John may take aspirin, NSAIDs, drink, or smoke; Bill may be into living organically and never put an impure thing into his body, whether medication or cigarettes. Both Bill and John can be infected with *H. pylori*, but John is far more likely to develop an ulcer than Bill.

The strongest evidence that suggests *H. pylori* causes ulcers is that ulcers don't come back when *H. pylori* is treated.

There is also an ethical issue regarding treating asymptomatic people with antibiotics. Antibiotics can lead to resistant strains of bacteria.

Antibiotic Therapy

No single antibiotic appears to be effective in killing *H. pylori*. Therefore, what's known as "combination therapy" is often used, where a combination of two antibiotics, an H2 receptor antagonist and the antacid bismuth (the main ingredient in Pepto-Bismol) are prescribed together. Or two antibiotics with a proton inhibitor may be prescribed. It's believed that *H. pylori* has a variety of strains. The use of two antibiotic agents gives more of a guarantee that the right strain of *H. pylori* will be killed.

The best combination of antibiotics and ulcer drugs keeps changing as newer studies are released.

Take only "as prescribed"

Recently, several national campaigns in a variety of countries have been funded to teach people how to take antibiotics. That's because antibiotics are dangerous—not to you, but to the future of the human race. The more antibiotics that are prescribed, the more potential there is for them to be misused, which leads to resistant strains of bacteria that no antibiotic can cure. Studies show that antibiotics are also misprescribed in a variety of scenarios; patients may insist on antibiotics for a viral infection, for example, when antibiotics, by definition, can treat only bacteria, not viruses. Studies show that 70 percent of patients insist on prescriptions for antibiotics for viral infections; many doctors give in rather than argue. Antibiotics are also requested as "preventive" medicine to ward off feared bacteria. This is not what antibiotics were designed to do. Unfortunately, when people take them as "prevention pills," other friendly bacteria in the body have a chance to mutate.

The biggest problem is that people don't understand how antibiotics work, and therefore they stop taking them as soon as they feel well. This does not allow the antibiotic to kill all the bacteria it was meant to kill, and it allows the bacteria time to mutate and resist that antibiotic.

Shockingly, more than 50 percent of people in one survey failed to take their antibiotics as prescribed—even though 75 percent of those surveyed said that they were counseled about how to take the medication.

Contributing factors to the problem are antibiotics prescribed in pediatric medicine. Antibiotics prescribed each year for the roughly 24.5 million children's ear infections in the United States can also lead to resistant strains of bacteria.

Therefore, it's crucial that you follow these directions whenever an antibiotic is prescribed:

1. Take your antibiotic as prescribed (for example, with meals, or at night). Don't take four pills a day when you're supposed to take one; don't take it once a day when you're supposed to take it three times a day. In other words, be sure you understand how many pills to take each day and when to take them. Skipping doses can allow the antibiotic to become ineffective, and give your bacteria some time to mutate. Doubling up on a dose is usually not encouraged, either.

2. Ask how alcohol, milk, or other foods will affect the antibiotic. Some foods can weaken the antibiotic and make it ineffective.

3. FINISH THE BOTTLE. Don't stop taking the antibiotic because you feel better. You're feeling better because the bacteria may be dying; but they are not completely "dead" until the bottle is finished. Many antibiotics must be taken several times a day for ten or more days to do the job, even though you will probably feel better within forty-eight hours.

4. Never take "leftover" antibiotics from a prescription you didn't finish last year. And never borrow an antibiotic from your sister-in-law's friend's mother, or lend it to your brother's friend's sister-in-law!

5. Be prepared for some side effects. Antibiotics kill off friendly bacteria in your body, too, and classically they cause vaginal yeast infections. You may also experience nausea, diarrhea, rashes, or a number of other side effects. Ask your doctor what to expect before you fill your prescription. Antibiotics may also affect other medications you're taking and render them ineffective. Oral contraceptives and antibiotics don't mix, for example. You may wind up trading an ulcer for a baby if you're not careful.

What happens if I don't take my antibiotic correctly?

Hospitals all over the world are seeing mutated bacteria that nothing can kill. People are dying of diseases that used to be treatable. If people don't become more responsible about antibiotics, resistant strains of bacteria may outpace the development of new drugs to kill them. Because we have so many antibiotics around, many pharmaceutical companies have been focusing on antifungals and antiviral medications instead.

The Centers for Disease Control estimate that about forty thousand Americans die each year due to antibiotic-resistant strains of bacteria. For more information on the consequences of not taking your drugs "as prescribed," pick up a copy of *The Antibiotic Paradox,* by Dr. Stuart Levy, a professor at Tufts Medical School.

If you had a gastric (or duodenal) ulcer that was complicated, it's important to see your doctor six to eight weeks after your ulcer has healed to make sure that you are indeed ulcer-free. It's also important to make sure that what you had was in fact an ulcer and not a cancerous lesion. As discussed earlier in this chapter, cancer can sometimes be mistaken for an ulcer. It's also important to keep in mind that just because you have been treated for an ulcer, you are not immune to other gastrointestinal problems, such as GERD, discussed next.

CHAPTER 4

WHEN THE ISSUE IS NUD AND GERD

If you've just read chapter 2, and your doctor has told you that your pain and heartburn symptoms do not sound like an ulcer, you've come to the right place! Non-ulcer dyspepsia (NUD), or "hmmm, discomfort not due to ulcer," is not a disease; it is simply an umbrella term that helps doctors distinguish ulcer patients from non-ulcer patients. When a doctor tells you that you have NUD, it's like telling a person with a runny nose and tearing eyes that her symptoms are due to "non-cold virus discomfort" when, in fact, she has an allergy. In other words, it sounds "medical" but it is not a clear-cut diagnosis that should satisfy you. This chapter discusses the disorders that fall under NUD: gastroesophageal reflux disease (GERD) and dysmotility (meaning "gastrointestinal tract muscles not moving very well"). The symptoms, diagnosis, and treatment of GERD and dysmotility are the focus of this chapter.

WHEN IT ISN'T AN ULCER
BUT IT FEELS LIKE ONE

Gastroenterologists explain the typical NUD patient as someone who has symptoms that are completely indistinguishable from signs of ulcers and heartburn, but whose stomach and esophagus look completely normal in diagnostic tests. In these cases, it's believed that there is an underlying disorder at work called dysmotility, where the muscles of the GI tract are not as coordinated as they should be. Therefore, while you may have an "acid problem," the problem is not that you have too much acid, but rather, you have acid in the wrong place. Dysmotility is diagnosed when there are a few symptoms in addition to pain and heartburn: bloating, difficulty finishing a meal (aka early satiety), gas, and/or nausea. Other symptoms that fall into the dysmotility arena include a general feeling of stomach discomfort during or after eating, and the need to belch, but most people will notice the first group of symptoms. People with dysmotility will find that antacid medications don't work very well, including H2 receptor antagonists. That's because acid-suppressing drugs cannot fix the underlying motility problem.

Sometimes the term *ulcerlike* is used to describe symptoms of NUD. In this case, reflux is not the problem; pain and discomfort are. But again, no ulcer will be present. Experts believe that people who have ulcerlike symptoms without reflux may also have dysmotility. Symptoms of NUD can, in fact, be so "gray" that many doctors essentially flip a coin to decide what to rule out by prescribing a short course of drug therapy to see what happens. In other words, people with NUD will either respond to a particular medication or not; the response will tell the doctor whether that person has GERD or dysmotility, or both.

What Exactly Is Gastroesophageal Reflux Disease (GERD)?

GERD is a confusing disease consisting of chronic heartburn/reflux (see chapter 2), as well as many dysmotility symptoms such as bloating and nausea. One survey showed that 75 percent of people suffering from non-ulcer pain and heartburn have additional symptoms. As discussed in chapter 2, reflux is caused when the lower esophageal sphincter (LES)—the muscle connecting the esophagus with the stomach—doesn't close properly after food passes from the esophagus to the stomach. So acid-laced food comes back up.

In the medical community, GERD is referred to as an "iceberg" disease because there are many symptoms at the base common to all people with GERD. As the iceberg narrows into various jagged peaks, there are variations in the symptoms. For example, all people will have reflux, but not all will feel the burning, bloating, or nausea. On the other hand, other people may experience every imaginable symptom of GERD and dysmotility. Moreover, the severity of the symptoms will differ, depending on how severe LES dysfunction is, how much fluid is coming up from the stomach, and even how effective saliva is at neutralizing the reflux. Most experts today classify GERD as both an acid problem (in that acid is in the wrong part of the GI tract) and a motility problem.

However, GERD can also exist with normal motility. For example, GERD occurs during pregnancy as a perfectly natural discomfort. In this case, the top of the uterus pushes up the GI tract, while progesterone relaxes many of the body's muscles, including the LES. Some doctors believe a hiatal hernia may weaken the LES and cause GERD. See chapter 7 for more details.

An esophageal ulcer

When GERD is severe, an ulcer can develop in the lining of the esophagus. In this case, the ulcer is caused by acid in an area where it doesn't belong. *H. pylori* is not considered a culprit in these ulcers. About 5 percent of all ulcers are of this type. It's more common for severe GERD to cause inflammation of the esophageal lining, which is known as esophagitis. This can lead to narrowing of the esophagus. (When the esophagus is inflamed, it narrows, just like shoes become suddenly too tight when your feet expand.)

When You Have Dysmotility

As discussed in chapter 1, food travels from the esophagus into the stomach, which slowly releases it into the small intestine. There can be problems on any or all "floors" of this elevator. The lower esophageal sphincter relaxes when it should be taut, allowing food to come back up. Or, things can get stuck between the stomach and small intestine, which causes the symptoms of bloating, fullness, and so on. (See Table 4.1.)

Dysmotility, with all of its varying symptoms, is typically a chronic condition. Symptoms keep coming back, and by the time dysmotility is finally diagnosed, most people have had these symptoms for a long time. The only way you can stop symptoms from recurring is by changing your life-style habits or taking a motility drug as a "maintenance" drug. (See further on.)

Diagnosing dysmotility

Many people with a motility disorder will be misdiagnosed. One reason is that most diagnostic tests will come back normal when there is a motility problem. As discussed in chapter 2, most of the diagnostic tests available for GI disorders are for the purpose of ruling out an ulcer, tumor, or inflammation.

The classic case of dysmotility goes something like this: You may notice that you suffer from chronic gas, bloating, and feeling full despite your efforts to control it. You may also have

TABLE 4.1   **Is It an Ulcer or Dysmotility?**

Sounds like an ulcer if:	Sounds like dysmotility if:	See a specialist if:
you notice that . . .	*you have some or all of . . .*	*you are 40+ and/or suddenly notice . . .*
hunger-pang pain wakes you up	heartburn	it's hard to swallow
pain is relieved by food or antacids	reflux	weight loss
you can pinpoint pain	belching or gas	black stools
you've had an ulcer before	bloating and/or nausea and/or pain after eating	bloody saliva
you're taking aspirin or NSAIDs	pain is hard to pinpoint	bloody vomit
there's a family history of ulcer	symptoms are not relieved by antacids	chest pain
you smoke	symptoms don't wake you up at night	cough/asthma
you have black stools or bloody vomit		no therapy helps

Source: Adapted from physician literature, Janssen-Ortho, Inc., 1996.

a lot of stress in your life combined with poor eating habits. Your doctor had prescribed H2 receptor antagonists (e.g., Tagamet), but they didn't help. You were then sent for tests, which came back normal. You were also counseled about changing your diet and life-style to avoid symptoms, but you're not very good at making dietary changes. Your symptoms persist and you're miserable. Several months later, another doctor (perhaps a GI specialist) diagnoses a motility disorder, prescribes a specific motility drug or prokinetic agent, which may help your symptoms disappear.

Dysmotility is often missed because doctors tend to think of ulcers or reflux when they're diagnosing upper GI disorders. Many times, lesser symptoms such as gas or bloating are not reported. Chapter 2 devotes significant space to properly reporting your symptoms in the first place. Sometimes people have suffered from dysmotility symptoms for so long, they don't think of their symptoms as abnormal or worthy of reporting. That's why it's crucial to review the section in chapter 2 on what your doctor should ask you.

MOVING RIGHT ALONG

Most gastroenterologists agree that making certain life-style adjustments can probably clear up GERD and restore motility without the use of drug therapy. That said, we know from diabetes studies that only about 8 percent of the population can actually make the necessary changes to improve overall diet and health. Chapter 9 discusses in more detail how to eat right and feel better.

But even if you cannot change your dietary habits, you can improve gravity. Experts recommend elevating the head of your bed by placing 6-inch blocks under the mattress, which will minimize the heartburn/reflux symptoms.

Drugs That Make Things Go

If you suffer from bloating, feeling full, and the symptoms that comprise dysmotility along with heartburn and pain, then you don't need an acid-suppressing drug or an H2 receptor antagonist. What you need in this case is a prokinetic drug that will improve motility and get things moving again. Right now, the most common prokinetic drug on the market is cisapride (Propulsid in the United States; Prepulsid in Canada). Cisapride regulates the muscles in the GI tract by telling the brain to send the right "messages" to the muscles that control the GI tract. Those muscles include the lower esophageal sphincter, which will stop relaxing when it should be contracting. In essence, cisapride helps food get from the esophagus into the stomach, and then from the stomach into the small intestine. It does this by improving LES pressure and peristalsis, which gets rid of the acid in the esophagus and improves gastric emptying. Once that happens, you'll notice that all the symptoms caused by food sitting around in your stomach too long will disappear. Older prokinetic drugs include bethanechol and metoclopramide, but they're not used very often anymore.

What about acid suppressants?

Only 5 to 10 percent of all GERD sufferers are in fact secreting too much stomach acid. Once the lower esophageal sphincter delivers food into the stomach and squeezes shut like it's supposed to do, acid-laced food will no longer come back up into the esophagus. No more half-digested food, no more reflux or heartburn, and, therefore, no more need to use antacids or H2 receptor antagonists.

In cases where severe reflux has caused esophagitis or an ulcer, an H2 receptor drug such as cimetidine, famotidine, nizatidine, or ranitidine can help to alleviate acid symptoms until cisapride starts to work its magic. Many doctors in this case will instead prescribe one of the proton pump inhibitors, such as omeprazole, lansoprazole, or pantoprazole (in Canada only), which inhibits an enzyme necessary for acid secretion. If you have only mild reflux, then regular over-the-counter antacids, combined with cisapride, may help. However, in most cases of GERD, the acid is simply in the wrong spot—something an acid-lowering drug cannot do much about.

How long does it take for these medications to work?

If you have esophagitis, you won't begin to feel completely better until the lining of your esophagus has healed, which can take about three months. Everybody has some acid that normally gets into the esophagus. Once it's irritated, however, the esophagus will be more sensitive so that even normal amounts of acid could cause some symptoms while you're taking your medication. It's also important to try to adjust your eating habits while you're on medications, cutting out many of the "trigger" foods discussed in chapter 9, as well as refraining from bad habits such as eating large meals before bedtime.

What If Symptoms Persist?

If your symptoms of dysmotility and GERD are not getting better with cisapride alone or in combination with other drugs, that's alarming. In this case, your doctor should do further diagnostic tests to investigate *why* you're not getting better.

As discussed in chapter 2, an upper GI series can shed some light on what's going on in your esophagus in terms of swallowing, as well as show how well your stomach is emptying. The scrambled egg test, mentioned in chapter 2, can also help to document the time it takes for the esophagus to clear out the radioactive tracer, which will help your doctor to understand a little more about esophageal clearing. This test may also provide information on how quickly your stomach empties both solids and liquids.

For this test, a nuclear medicine technician will play "chef," and prepare scrambled eggs for you with technetium (a radioactive substance) as a tracer. You'll eat the eggs and then a gamma counter will be placed over your stomach after you've swallowed to "follow" the eggs on their journey through your GI tract. The test should determine how quickly the eggs leave your stomach.

These tests should only be done after ulcers, esophagitis, and tumors have been ruled out through endoscopy.

Many gastroenterologists believe, however, that there are no good tests to check gastric emptying or motility. If your gastroenterologist comes from this school, then he or she may decide to try a combination of drugs to see how well you respond. Atypical symptoms may warrant pH testing or manometry, discussed in chapter 2.

Certain tests need to be done properly in order to extract any useful information. For example, people who have difficulty swallowing need to be investigated for some sort of obstacle or obstruction in the esophagus. In this case, imaging tests need to be done while you're in various positions, when the most stress is placed on the esophagus. Imaging tests should be done while you're upright as well as lying down. It's also useful to have an imaging test done after you've had a soft drink, so your doctor can have a good look at the stomach when it's "ballooning" out.

If your symptoms persist despite treatment, and all other serious diseases (such as cancer) have been ruled out, then you may require surgery. In this case, a procedure known as fundoplication can be done to physically increase the pressure in the lower esophagus. This is definitely a last-resort approach that should not be done unless all treatment options have been tried.

HOW TO KEEP GERD FROM COMING BACK

One of the biggest problems with treating GERD is dealing with relapse. GERD has a bad habit of returning as soon as you stop your medication unless you make some dramatic life-style changes, discussed in chapter 9.

That's because cisapride does not permanently repair GI motility; it restores it while you're taking the drug. Your doctor may therefore recommend a lower maintenance dose of cisapride to be taken once your initial symptoms have disappeared. This greatly depends on the severity of your condition and your doctor's philosophy regarding relapse. If you have severe esophagitis (severe ulcers or a narrowing of the esophagus), you may be prescribed a proton pump inhibitor such as omeprazole for long-term maintenance. Many gastroenterologists swear by this method.

How fast your symptoms return also has to do with whether you're taking your medication as prescribed. The more pills you take in a day, the more room there is for missing pills, which could cause your symptoms to return.

If you've had mild GERD, you may not need to be on any maintenance therapy other than an occasional antacid or an H2 receptor drug as needed.

The Recipe for Prevention

The vast majority of people with GERD will reexperience symptoms as soon as they stop their medications. This can occur within a few weeks or within six months. In fact, 85 to 90 percent of all people with GERD will experience relapse. The problem with any treatment for GERD is that the medication is designed to fix things only as long as you're taking it. There are no good studies that can definitely say: "When you combine drug A with drug B, you can prevent GERD from recurring." As a result, many doctors combine certain therapies based on what they've seen in their own practice; there are no rules, in other words. Some doctors may have a lot of success by combining cisapride with an H2 receptor drug, while others may find that solely using a proton pump inhibitor is a better way to prevent relapse. The problem with most drug studies is that they are short-term studies, which are not useful in this instance.

The best approach to preventing relapse is to make some lifestyle changes once your initial symptoms are healed. If that doesn't work, some sort of ongoing medication may be prescribed on an intermittent basis or daily. What you take and how much you take largely depends on how well you've responded to various medications in the past and your own feelings about taking a maintenance drug. Maintenance therapy may include cisapride, an H2 receptor drug, or a proton pump inhibitor, used in people who have had very severe symptoms.

Relapse vs. incorrect therapy

Many people with recurring GERD were never treated appropriately to begin with. For example, people who have dysmotility symptoms along with heartburn and reflux will usually find relief with cisapride because that's the drug that restores motility to the upper GI tract. If you've been prescribed only acid-lowering or suppressing drugs, your dysmotility was never addressed. So in this case, your "relapse" is really a case of symptoms persisting despite treatment. Experts agree that the majority of people who are put on an H2 receptor drug and then have recurrent or persisting symptoms within a couple of weeks, have dysmotility and should be prescribed a prokinetic drug instead of an acid-lowering drug. But some people may need *both* drugs if they have GERD and dysmotility.

Maintenance dosages

If you've been prescribed cisapride, you'll probably be instructed to take a 20-mg pill twice a day. Once symptoms subside, you'll probably be given a 10-mg pill twice a day to prevent relapse. If

you seem to suffer from symptoms at night and wake up nause-
ated, you may be prescribed a 20-mg pill at bedtime. If you're
doing shift work and seem to suffer from GERD only when
you're working odd-hour shifts, then it's fine to take cisapride as
needed.

H2 receptor drugs will usually be prescribed for maintenance
dosing at 800 mg at bedtime or 600 mg twice daily, while proton pump inhibitors such as omeprazole will be prescribed at 20
mg daily. See chapter 5 for more information about dosages and
side effects.

What About *H. Pylori*?

As discussed in the previous chapter, *H. pylori* is a bacteria that is
believed to cause peptic ulcer disease. Like GERD, ulcers had a
very high relapse rate until the discovery of *H. pylori,* which
proved that ulcer disease was of infectious origin. About 95 to
100 percent of people with duodenal ulcer disease (who are not
taking aspirin or NSAIDs) are infected with *H. pylori*; approxi-
mately 65 percent of people with gastric ulcers are infected with
H. pylori. It's been shown that by treating *H. pylori* in people with
ulcers, the recurrence rate drops significantly. Roughly 90 percent
of all people who are treated for *H. pylori* will never have an ulcer
again. This remarkable phenomenon has raised the question of
whether *H. pylori* is a factor in GERD. Should it be treated? The
answer at this stage of the game is "sometimes."

Until quite recently, there has been no indication for screening people for *H. pylori* who have non-ulcer conditions. However, a recent panel on the question has decided that in "select"
cases of NUD or GERD, treating *H. pylori* has been of some benefit. It remains to be seen whether these benefits are:

- ▣ **coincidental** (John Doe stopped eating chili burgers the week he was put on antibiotics for *H. pylori* infection; it was really the chili burger that was the problem);
- ▣ **placebo effect** (the belief that *H. pylori* is a factor in his illness causes John Doe to get better); or
- ▣ **real** (it turns out that inflammation triggered by John Doe's *H. pylori* did, indeed, induce a motility problem).

We just don't know which possibility is the correct answer. If your doctor decides to treat *H. pylori* to prevent GERD relapse, read the section on antibiotics in the previous chapter.

Life-style modification, again, can be a very effective way of managing GERD. Nevertheless, the majority of patients will be taking some form of medication to control symptoms. Everything you need to know "About Those Stomach Medicines"—whether they're over-the-counter or prescribed—is discussed in the next chapter.

CHAPTER 5

ABOUT THOSE STOMACH MEDICINES

T his chapter is the one to read if you're in the habit of taking antacids or have been prescribed a potent acid-lowering/ controlling drug or a prokinetic drug. While over-the-counter antacids tend to be eaten like candy, contrary to popular belief, they're not intended for long-term use. Meanwhile, many prescription drugs, such as cisapride, are taken on an "as needed" basis, even though this is not how the drug was designed to be used. What you need to know about usage, side effects, and other drugs known to irritate the GI tract—drugs that are not stomach medications—are discussed in this chapter. Drugs used to treat bowel disorders are discussed in chapter 6.

DROPPING ANTACIDS

If you walk down the "stomach aisle" of any drugstore, you'll find a dizzying variety of antacids (such as Tums and Rolaids) and what are called acid-lowering drugs, acid-controlling drugs or, more to the point, acid-blocking drugs. These are the stronger drugs discussed in previous chapters, known as H2 receptor antagonists (cimetidine, famotidine, nizatidine, and ranitidine). Until recently, all H2 receptor antagonists were prescription drugs. In the United States, you can now purchase these drugs in an over-the-counter formulation, which contains a lower dosage than the prescription version. Pepcid and Tagamet are examples of over-the-counter H2 receptor antagonists. (Tagamet still requires a prescription in Canada.) We often make the assumption that if something is sold over-the-counter, it can be taken every day, any time. *This is not the case.* If you read the labels, the manufacturers will tell you so. Antacids are intended for mild bouts of heartburn. Unfortunately, many people take them every day. If this is your case, see your doctor to find out what's causing this chronic condition.

Antacids

Antacids relieve heartburn (also known as acid indigestion or sour stomach) as well as peptic ulcer disease symptoms (see chapter 3) by neutralizing the stomach acid that rises into the esophagus. Various neutralizing agents can work on hydrochloric acid (stomach acid). For example, some brands contain aluminum hydroxide (e.g., Amphojel); some brands contain calcium carbonate (e.g., Tums or Rolaids); some brands contain magnesium (e.g., Mylanta or Maalox); and some brands use the foaming agent alginic acid. Foamy antacids are thought to work because the foam seems to form a barrier between the stomach and esophagus, preventing heartburn in some people.

An interesting variant (which doesn't contain alginic acid) is the ever-popular Alka-Seltzer. This common antacid actually contains three principal ingredients: aspirin, sodium bicarbonate, and citric acid, which in water forms sodium citrate and sodium acetylsalicylate. That's a lot of medication. And if you read the label, Alka-Seltzer is indicated for heartburn *combined* with headache and/or aches and pains from "overindulgence in food and drink." (Not surprisingly, Alka-Seltzer is a popular hangover cure.)

How long can you take them?

All antacids allow a maximum number of tablets or teaspoons per day that is fairly liberal. For example, you can take up to sixteen Tums per day. You're allowed eight tablets of Alka-Seltzer per day. If you prefer a liquid form of antacid, you're allowed sixteen teaspoons of Maalox or Gaviscon per day. But you can't do this forever. All antacid labels explicitly say something akin to "Consult your physician if symptoms persist beyond two weeks." This means that your romance with antacids has to end after two weeks; if you take the maximum daily dosage every day for a period that exceeds two weeks, you could suffer from the following side effects:

- diarrhea
- problems metabolizing calcium
- a buildup of magnesium, which can aggravate or trigger kidney disease (particularly in people who have diabetes)
- possible lead toxicity (currently, an environmental group is in the process of suing makers of various antacid and calcium supplements, alleging that their products contain dangerous amounts of lead)

Many antacids cannot be combined with the antibiotic tetracycline or with anticoagulants, such as warfarin. It's always best to check with a pharmacist before you purchase the product.

Acid Blockers

If you have chronic heartburn or reflux, your doctor may prescribe an H2 receptor antagonist, which is different from an antacid. These medications actually inhibit the stomach from secreting acid in the first place. The four H2 receptor antagonists on the market now are cimetidine (Tagamet), famotidine (Pepcid), nizatidine (Axid), and ranitidine (Zantac). In the United States, all these drugs are sold over-the-counter at lower strengths than the dosages available in prescription form. In Canada, only Pepcid is over-the-counter.

H2 antagonists are always prescribed when an ulcer is diagnosed or when someone suffers from gastroesophageal reflux disease and can be used to heal ulcers and esophagitis. They are usually recommended for short-term rather than long-term use. However, if you respond well to an acid-blocking drug, many doctors will recommend that you continue to take it as maintenance therapy for a prolonged period of anywhere from six to twelve months. That's because H2 receptor drugs are considered to be fairly safe drugs that are relatively cheap, with an easy dosing schedule of one or two tablets per day. If your symptoms don't improve with continued use of an H2 receptor drug, it often means that you have a motility problem and/or a more complicated acid problem.

If you have symptoms of dysmotility (see chapter 4), an H2 receptor antagonist is probably not the drug for you; in this case, you need a motility or prokinetic agent such as cisapride, discussed further on. In fact, many people will take an H2 receptor drug repeatedly without seeing their symptoms dissipate.

Dosages and length of therapy

In the early 1980s, the American Medical Association recommended that H2 receptor drugs be used for a period of two weeks to initially treat the symptoms, and then for an additional four weeks to prevent symptoms from coming back. No doctor follows these dosing guidelines anymore. If you're not responding to H2 receptor drugs within a couple of weeks, your doctor will prescribe either a motility drug or an extremely potent acid-lowering drug, known as a proton pump inhibitor, such as omeprazole (Prilosec or Losec) or lansoprazole (Prevacid). These are available only by prescription. (See Table 5.1.)

TABLE 5.1 **What Therapy Should Be Used First When You Have Chronic Heartburn?**

Start by:

- Modifying your diet and life-style habits (see chapter 9) with or without over-the-counter antacids.

If you don't find relief, your doctor can prescribe one of the following:

- Prokinetic agent (cisapride)

- H2 receptor antagonist (cimetidine, famotidine, nizatidine, or ranitidine)

If you're still not finding relief, your doctor can prescribe:

- a proton pump inhibitor (omeprazole, lansoprazole)

or

- rule out a more serious condition with tests (see chapter 2)

Source: Adapted from J. C. Reynolds, "Individualized Acute Treatment Strategies for Gastroesophageal Reflux Disease." Scandinavian Journal of Gastroenterology 30, Suppl. 213 (1995): 17–24.

Dosages are all over the map, depending on which brand you're taking. For nizatidine, 150 mg is taken twice a day; prescription-strength cimetidine is taken at much higher doses (400 mg twice daily); famotidine is taken in one 40-mg tablet once a day; while ranitidine is taken as 300 mg once daily or 150 mg twice daily. See Tables 5.2, 5.3, and 5.4 for the list of common side effects of each of these drugs.

Drugs that cannot be combined with acid blockers

Cimetidine cannot be combined with the following drugs:

- anticoagulants, such as warfarin
- phenytoin
- propranolol
- chlordiazepoxide
- lidocaine
- diazepam
- theophylline
- nifedipine

If you're taking any of the above medications, you can request famotidine or nizatidine. Ranitidine, specifically, cannot be combined with NSAIDs, theophylline, or oral hypoglycemic agents.

DRUGS FOR MOTILITY PROBLEMS

When your doctor tells you that you have a motility problem—more specifically, dysmotility—it means that your stomach's motion is impaired. In this case, the acid is in the esophagus because the digestive tract's muscles are not coordinating well enough for the lower esophagus sphincter to work (see chapters 2 and 4). Prokinetic drugs are prescribed for dysmotility symptoms; these are symptoms such as bloating and inability to finish a meal, which accompany pain and heartburn. Prokinetic drugs, as discussed in chapter 4, work by restoring proper motility to the digestive tract's muscles. The problem with prokinetic drugs is that many people don't take them as prescribed. When that happens, the drugs are not dangerous in any way, but they won't work.

The most common prokinetic drug is cisapride (Propulsid;

TABLE 5.2   **Side Effects of Prokinetic Drugs**

1. Metoclopramide	2. Domperidone	3. Cisapride
drowsiness (10%)	dry mouth (1.9%)	diarrhea (5.1%)
fatigue (10%)	headache/migraine (1.2%)	stomach cramps (2.1%)
lassitude (10%)		headache (1.6%)
insomnia (5%)	gastrointestinal (2.4%)	vertigo/dizziness (1.2%)
headache (5%)	endocrinological (1.3%): hot flushes,	
dizziness (5%)	mastalgia,	
bowel disturbances (5%)	galactorrhea, gynecomastia,	
galactorrhea	and/or menstrual irregularities	
menstrual disorders		
parkinsonism		
increases in prolactin		

Sources: 1. Maxeran product monograph. 2. Motilium product monograph.
3. Prepulsid product monograph.

Prepulsid in Canada). Other prokinetic drugs are metoclopramide (Maxeran) and domperidone (Motilium, Canada only). Cisapride is the newest prokinetic drug, while metoclopramide and domperidone are considered to be older generations of prokinetic drugs. One gastroenterologist describes cisapride as a drug that "puts the foot on the accelerator," while the other two prokinetic drugs "take the foot off the brake." In other words, pressing on the gas will get you farther, faster, than just "not braking." In addition, about 25 percent of people on metoclopramide and 8 percent of those on domperidone will experience embarrassing side effects, such as breast enlargement (that goes for men, too) and even lactation. In fact, domperidone is frequently prescribed

TABLE 5.3   **Side Effects of Proton Pump Inhibitors**
The following side effects were reported in at least 1 percent of people taking the drug.

Omeprazole	Lansoprazole
Headache	Headache
Diarrhea	Diarrhea
Nausea	Abdominal pain
Upper respiratory infection	Nausea
Dizziness	Dizziness
Vomiting	Rash
Rash	
Constipation	
Cough	
Back pain	

Source: Prilosec patient information, February 1997; Prevacid product monograph, 1996.

to breast-feeding mothers to stimulate milk production. (You can read all about this in *The Breastfeeding Sourcebook*.) Table 5.2 compares the side effects of all three prokinetic drugs so you can get an idea of how well-tolerated cisapride is compared to the older agents. That said, many gastroenterologists find that different patients respond better to different prokinetic drugs. Cisapride will not work well for everyone! But in light of the fact that cisapride is really the only prokinetic drug that is currently prescribed, the remainder of this section will address cisapride only.

How Much for How Long?

Cisapride takes a while to work. That's because of the nature of the stomach problem—it's not emptying properly. In order to

TABLE 5.4   **Major Side Effects of H2 Receptor Antagonists**

1. Nizatidine *(in at least 1%)*	2. Famotidine *(in at least 1%)*	3. Ranitidine *(reported— % not cited)*	4. Cimetidine *(reported— % not cited)*
Sweating	Headache	Headache	Diarrhea
Somnolence	Dizziness	Malaise	Tiredness
Rash	Constipation	Dizziness	Dizziness
	Diarrhea	Somnolence	Skin rashes
	Nausea	Insomnia	Hair loss
		Vertigo	Confusion in elderly
		Constipation	
		Diarrhea	
		Nausea/vomiting	
		Abdominal pain	

Source: 1. Axid product monograph, 1996. 2. Pepcid product monograph, 1996. 3. Zantac product monograph, 1996. 4. Tagamet product monograph, 1997.

work, cisapride needs to be absorbed into the bloodstream once it leaves the stomach. Since your stomach is not emptying normally, it will take some time for cisapride to get to work.

Cisapride is usually prescribed for a period of four to twelve weeks, depending on how quickly you're responding to it and how serious your symptoms were to begin with. Most people start to feel better within about two weeks. On the other hand, some people have almost immediate relief within a couple of days, while people with severe motility problems may find that it takes about a month before they feel better.

Different doctors have different ways of dosing cisapride. One method is to prescribe a 10-mg tablet to be taken about a half hour before each meal so that the drug has time to take effect before you eat. (Some doctors may also have you take an additional 10 mg at bedtime.) Another method is to simply have you take a 20-mg tablet twice a day (say, morning and at bedtime). Most doctors prefer twice-a-day dosing because it's easier for you to remember. Depending on how well you do on cisapride, you may be counseled to take 20 mg per day as a maintenance dose to keep your symptoms at bay. That's because, as discussed in chapter 4, as soon as you go off cisapride, your stomach's motility impairment may reappear. The drug fixes the problem as long as you take it, but it is not a cure-all.

Can't I just take it when I feel like it?

If you've responded well to a course of therapy with cisapride (lasting anywhere from four to twelve weeks), many doctors will tell you that it's fine to take cisapride on a temporary basis every so often. For example, if your symptoms have returned while you're going through a particularly stressful stage in your life, you can take cisapride for a couple of weeks until your life calms down again. But cisapride is not like Tums or Rolaids; it's not designed as a pill to pop before you go out for Mexican or Thai food. Nevertheless, many doctors will tell you that it's okay to do this *once in a while* (in other words, it won't hurt you), but don't get in the habit.

Is It Safe?

Even though cisapride is a prescription drug, its safety profile is better than that of many over-the-counter drugs. For instance, far fewer drugs conflict with it, compared to common antacids or acid-blocking drugs. In fact, the only drugs that you shouldn't use with cisapride are antifungal drugs. Most antibiotics, blood thinners, and anything else are fine when combined with cisapride, although some studies show that cisapride should not be prescribed with erythromycin or clarithromycin. Cisapride is also considered safe for seniors and has been used, on occasion, to relieve severe pregnancy-related GERD. The general rule, however, is to refrain from using all drugs during pregnancy, including antacids (although Tums markets itself as a calcium supplement for pregnant and lactating women).

Only 2 percent of people on cisapride experience any side effects, and these are mild. The major problems reported are headaches, some abdominal cramping, and either loose, frequent stools (which, by the way, many people welcome after being bloated and constipated for several months), or diarrhea. This tends to settle down in a week or so; if it doesn't, lowering the dosage should make the problem disappear. See Table 5.2 for the complete list of side effects.

THE "NUCLEAR WEAPONS"

If antacids are the "water pistols," proton pump inhibitors such as omeprazole (Prilosec; Losec in Canada) or lansoprazole (Prevacid) are the "nuclear weapons." These are very potent acid-suppressing drugs, which are reserved for severe situations only. That means in order to take this drug you must have:

- severe peptic ulcer disease (see chapter 3);
- severe gastroesophageal reflux disease (see chapter 4);
- severe esophagitis (see chapter 4); or
- an esophageal ulcer (see chapters 3 and 4).

In order to be classified as someone with a severe disease, you would first have to *not* respond to milder drugs, such as H2 receptor drugs or cisapride. Proton pump inhibitors should never be used in the presence of alarm symptoms (see chapter 2) unless a more serious disease, such as cancer, has been ruled out. The dosage really depends on why you're taking the drug.

How Much for How Long?

Proton pump inhibitors are intended as a short-term therapy only. If you're taking omeprazole, for the first two weeks of therapy you may take one tablet four times per day, and then half that dosage for an additional two weeks. Proton pump inhibitors are generally not recommended for longer than four weeks unless there are special circumstances. Proton pump inhibitors are also expensive drugs, compared to H2 receptor drugs; omeprazole costs roughly U.S. $75 per month compared to U.S. $10 for cimetidine. Therefore, prescribing these drugs as a maintenance therapy is considered inappropriate from a cost standpoint if another drug will work just as well. Some experts describe proton pump inhibitors as "too good" a drug. In other words, once you go on the drug, it's hard to coax you off it because it does such a good job of relieving acid-related symptoms. The problem is that this type of drug is not meant to be taken for a long time.

Side Effects

There are many side effects to proton pump inhibitors, as well as several drug interactions. Table 5.3 lists the major side effects that occur in more than 1 percent of people on these drugs. As far as drug interactions, the problems are with medications prescribed for other chronic conditions. The best advice is to give your doctor and pharmacist a list of all the drugs you're currently taking to see if any of them conflict. Often, proton pump inhibitors are prescribed in combination with an antibiotic; this is fine, as long as you're not taking another medication that conflicts with that antibiotic.

DRUGS THAT ARE HARD TO DIGEST

Throughout this book, the issue of aspirin and nonsteroidal anti-inflammatory drugs (NSAIDs) causing peptic ulcer disease has been raised. However, several other medications can also affect the digestive system, particularly oral medications. (See Table 5.5.) Many of the problems have to do with people taking their medications incorrectly. For example, if you're supposed to take a drug on an empty stomach, and you take it with food, or vice versa, you may be in for some nausea or vomiting. The older you get, the more vulnerable you are to digestive upset with various medications.

If you have food allergies, such as lactose or gluten intolerance, you may also have problems; lactose and gluten are often added to pills or tablets for taste and consistency.

The Esophagus Effects

A common problem with any pills that need to be swallowed is that they can irritate the esophagus. This is particularly the case when you're having trouble swallowing a giant "horse pill." If the pill stays in the esophagus too long, it can release its chemicals (meant for the small intestine) into the esophagus and irritate its lining. This can cause ulcers, bleeding, tearing, or inflammation. As a result, you'll experience pain when you swallow liquid or solid food. You may also literally feel the tablet lodged in your throat (in this case, eat a hearty crust of bread to get it down). You may also feel a dull ache in your chest or shoulder (that means the pain has radiated into your shoulder; however, the pill isn't in your shoulder) after you take the irritating medication. People especially susceptible to these problems include anyone with:

- esophagitis
- scleroderma (hardening of the skin)
- achalasia (irregular muscle activity of the esophagus)
- stroke

How to swallow it

Experts recommend that you swallow your tablets in a standing position. If you're bedridden or confined to a chair, sitting upright is best. Prior to taking the pill, first swallow some liquid to lubricate your throat, then take the pill with a full glass of liquid. After you swallow the pill, wait at least fifteen minutes before you lie down to make sure the pill has safely made it past your esophagus.

Certain drugs can cause general heartburn or reflux, even if you've done everything in your power to swallow correctly. These drugs include heart and blood pressure-lowering medications. In this case, all you can do is wait for the symptoms to pass and avoid other heartburn triggers, discussed in chapter 2. You may also require specific heartburn medications if your other medication is causing heartburn. Also review chapter 9.

NSAIDs Again

If you're taking a nonsteroidal anti-inflammatory drug (NSAID), such as ibuprofen or naproxen, the lining of your stomach can become irritated. In fact, in the absence of the bacterial infection *H. pylori* (see chapter 3), NSAIDs and aspirin use are the most common causes of peptic ulcer disease.

NSAIDs work a little bit like *H. pylori* in that they can weaken the stomach lining's ability to resist its own acid. The older you are, the more at risk you are for NSAID-induced stomach irritations because you're more likely to be taking NSAIDs as pain relievers for arthritic conditions. Requesting coated tablets,

TABLE 5.5   **A Dozen Drugs That Can Irritate the GI System**

1. Acetaminophen (Tylenol, Panadol, and Datril)

2. Antibiotics: penicillin (Amoxil, Amcill, and Augmentin); clindamycin; cephalosporins (Keflex and Ceclor); tetracyclines (Minocin, Sumycin, and Vibramycin); quinolones (Cipro); sulfa drugs (Bactrim)

3. Anticholinergics: propantheline (Pro-Banthine) and dicyclomine (Bentyl); amitriptyline (Elavil and Endep); and nortriptyline (Aventyl and Pamelor); levodopa (Dopar), and carbidopa and levodopa combination (Sinemet)

4. Anticonvulsants: phenytoin (Dilantin) and valproic acid (Dalpro)

5. Antihypertensives: Warfarin

6. Calcium Channel Blockers: diltiazem (Cardizem); nifedipine (Procardia); and verapamil (Isoptin)

7. Chlorpromazine (Thorazine and Ormazine)

8. Colchicine

9. Nitrates: isosorbide dinitrate (Iso-Bid and Isonate) and nitroglycerin (Nitro-Bid and Nitrocap)

10. Nonsteroidal anti-inflammatory drugs (NSAIDs): aspirin (Bayer and Bufferin); ibuprofen (Advil, Nuprin, and Motrin); tomectin (Tolectin); naproxen (Naprosyn); and piroxicam (Feldene)

11. Quinidine: Quinalan and Quinaglute

12. Theophylline: Theo-Dur, Theophyl, and Bronkodyl

Source: Adapted from patient literature produced by the National Digestive Diseases Information Clearinghouse, 1994–1996.

avoiding alcohol, and taking your pills with milk or water can be somewhat helpful, but these measures don't always work.

Drugs That Cause Dysmotility

Anticholinergics (cholesterol-lowering drugs), antidepressants, and drugs used to treat Parkinson's disease are notorious for causing motility problems. In this case, there is no magic technique you can employ before, during, or after taking the drug to prevent dysmotility. The only remedy is switching to a different medication, or taking a motility agent such as cisapride along with the culprit medication.

Drugs That Cause Bowel Problems

The most common side effects of any medications are constipation and diarrhea. Constipation can be caused by any drug that affects the nerves and muscle activity in the colon. When this happens, stools are slow to come, and hard when they do come. Antihypertensives, anticholinergics, cholestyramine, iron, and aluminum-containing antacids are the most guilty offenders. Adjusting your diet and life-style is the only way to combat this problem. (I'll tell you what to do in chapter 9.) You can also take a laxative with your doctor's permission, or a stool softener can be prescribed.

As for diarrhea, antibiotics may cause this because they kill off bacteria that normally live in the colon—bacteria that are there for good reason. Without this friendly "bowel bacteria," the overgrowth of another bacteria, called *Clostridium difficile* (*C. difficile*), may flourish. (However, it's important to note that antibiotics don't always cause this to happen.) The most common cause for diarrhea is just an alteration of the normal flora without *C. difficile*. This diarrhea is usually mild and will resolve once you stop taking the drug. *C. difficile*–associated diarrhea is more severe and usually requires treatment with metronidazole. *C. difficile* is actually responsible for colitis (inflammation of the colon). In response, the colon secretes excess water, which is what makes the stools runny. If you're taking a lot of antibiotics (and do turn to chapter 3 for directions on taking antibiotics), you may want to request alternatives to ampicillin, clindamycin, and the cephalosporin class of drugs; these are the ones that cause the most problems. How do you treat antibiotic-related diarrhea or colitis? The punchline is: with *another* antibiotic (one that kills off *C. difficile*).

Some drugs cause diarrhea simply because they "make water" in the colon. In this case, there is no inflammation, just too much fluid in the colon. Drugs known to do this are colchicine and magnesium-containing antacids. And finally, laxatives will often cause diarrhea because people tend to overuse them or abuse them. In this case, permanent damage to the nerves and muscles of the colon will cause chronic diarrhea.

A Word About Misoprostol

Occasionally, the drug misoprostol is prescribed in cases where NSAIDs and/or aspirin have caused an ulcer. More commonly, however, misoprostol is prescribed "off label" to induce abortion, as well as to prevent hemorrhaging after childbirth. It would never be prescribed during pregnancy, but if you think you might be pregnant, make sure you disclose this to your doctor before filling a prescription for misoprostol.

The next chapter is devoted to the final resting place of all things ingested, be it food, drink, or drug. The lower intestine is host to a myriad of disorders that leave millions of people frustrated, uncomfortable, and, consequently, well-read!

CHAPTER 6

BOWELS OF THE EARTH

One night my husband and I were invited to watch a video rental at the home of friends, among several other couples with whom we were only casually acquainted. The video was *Dumb and Dumber* (the title says it all!). In one of the dumber scenes, one of the characters unwittingly overdoses on a laxative and is seized with diarrhea at a most inopportune time. No noise was spared in the sound effects department. That was it for me; I was seized with a fit of uncontrollable laughter for the rest of the film. I laughed so hard my eyes were tearing and I couldn't catch my breath. The other couples in the room just looked at me in disdain and wonder; my husband was mortified. But how could I admit to them that I find nothing funnier than bathroom humor? How could I admit that my sister and I would, as children, sit outside the bathroom door and giggle to the sounds of flatulence made by our various relatives from the "old country." Clearly, I am not alone. No other part of the body is the source of more jokes, innuendo, or embarrassment than the lower GI tract. This fact makes it all the more difficult for people who suffer from bowel problems to report their symptoms to their doctor, or even to admit their symptoms to family members.

This chapter discusses the various bowel problems people are prone to, ranging from constipation, gas, infectious diarrhea, and irritable bowel syndrome (IBS), to the more serious conditions such as inflammatory bowel diseases (IBD), consisting of ulcerative colitis and Crohn's disease.

SIGNS OF INTELLIGENT LIFE

There's a wonderful children's book called *Everybody Poops*, by Taro Gomi. It teaches the reader that bowel movements, complete with noises and smells, come in all shapes, sizes, and shades. In fact, one of the most fascinating zoo experiences I ever had was watching a rhinoceros move its bowels before an awestruck crowd. It was like watching a live birth.

Small children will feel immediate pride in their bowel movements, and take cheerful delight in the gas noises they pass. In fact, babies who are not yet talking will suddenly become quite gleeful and excited after a bowel movement, laughing and jumping up and down; to most parents, this is a sign that the diaper needs to be changed! As we become adults, we learn to contain these feelings of glee, and we forget how satisfying normal, regular bowel movements are—*until they're gone*. So before I discuss all the various problems people experience in the lower GI tract, it's important to cover what constitutes *normal* bowel habits.

An Unremarkable Bowel

As discussed in chapter 1, the colon essentially acts as a solid waste container, drying out the waste that doesn't get absorbed further up. The nervous system controls the muscular contractions of the colon, which slowly move waste downward toward the rectum. We experience these stronger muscular contractions as the urge to have a bowel movement. Once we feel the urge, we sit down, relax, and allow the gentle contractions to overtake us. All we have to do is relax and the anal sphincter will open to allow the passage of stool.

The frequency of bowel movements varies from person to person. It's normal to move your bowels anywhere from a few times per day to a few times per week. A normal stool is solid or "formed" but not hard, and certainly should not contain mucus or blood. The stools should pass without cramps, pain, or strain. However, normal stools can pass noisily, since natural gas (called flatus)—swallowed air (nitrogen) that gets trapped in the lower intestine—often comes out with the stools, or independently. This is absolutely normal.

That smell

Here's a news flash: *People smell.* Just because it smells unpleasant, it doesn't mean it is not normal and natural. That goes for underarm odor, breath, sweat, vaginal odor, foot odor, urine, feces, and gas. Our body odors, or the odors of our bodily "products," are usually caused by bacteria (vaginal and foot odor are frequently caused by fungus).

The colon is swimming with friendly bacteria, which enjoy feasting on certain foods we eat, particularly legumes (beans and lentils) and cruciferous vegetables. A high-starch diet is also a culprit, where the nonabsorbable starches get sent to the colon and are eaten by bacteria. The more feasting these bacteria do, the more they excrete in the form of hydrogen sulfide and hydrocarbons. When this happens, you have more gas. The more sulfide gases that are generated by the bacteria, the smellier your gas or stools (that "rotten egg" smell).

When you have excessive flatulence

There's an old joke: A man tells his doctor that he suffers from continual "silent flatulence" and doesn't know what to do. In response, his doctor says: "The first thing we must do is check your hearing!" In other words, being aware of the problem is the first step in managing it.

Excessive flatulence is known as *lepetomania,* and is not considered a disease any more than halitosis (bad breath) is. Excessive gas (both odorless and malodorous), like bad breath, is certainly embarrassing but nothing to worry about. The cause is often related to diet (eating too much of a certain gas-producing food) or certain habits, such as gum-chewing or gulping air, which introduce too much nitrogen from the air into the GI tract, so that the gas comes out the other end. Gas is only a problem when it *doesn't* pass. In this case, you'll suffer from abdominal pain, distention, bloating, and often constipation.

Constipation

It's perfectly normal to experience occasional bouts of constipation. Constipation means that you are not experiencing an urge to move your bowels, and when you do, the stools are hard and difficult to pass. Generally, if more than three days have passed since your last bowel movement, the stools will harden. The colon will continue to dry out the stools because that's what the colon does. Before you say, "I'm constipated," remember that you don't need to have a bowel movement every day. Again, some people normally move their bowels only once or twice a week.

Most constipation is "functional" in that there is no disease or organic problem at work; it's a life-style problem, having to do with ignoring the urge to go (if you're surrounded by public toilets, for example), or not allowing enough time in the morning to create the urge to go by eating something. If you ignore the urge too often, you may stop feeling an urge altogether.

The worst thing you can do for occasional constipation is to run to the nearest laxative; this can create a dependency on laxatives, creating a merry-go-round of diarrhea-constipation-diarrhea cycles. Worse, your intestines can become so dependent on laxatives that they cannot work without them.

Few people, in fact, truly need a laxative for functional constipation. What they often need is simply enough time in the morning to eat something and to stay home for a little while until the urge comes. Adjusting the diet is an important factor in preventing constipation (see chapter 9). If you're contemplating a laxative, fiber or an osmatic laxative are preferable as they tend to be far gentler on your system. Some herbs, such as cascara sagrada, are considered more of a tonic than a laxative, and are said not to create a dependency, but cascara is still considered a stimulant laxative (see chapter 8).

There is also a myth that constipation is bad for your health. Diarrhea is far worse for your health. In fact, people never die from constipation, but they can from diarrhea. Colons are built to store stool. Nothing will happen to you if you don't move your bowels as regularly as you would like.

Other causes of constipation

Occasional constipation can also be caused by the following:

- Travel (changes in schedule, diet, and time zones can interfere with regularity)
- Hormonal imbalances/changes (e.g., an underactive thyroid gland or pregnancy)
- Anal sores (this includes fissures, hemorrhoids, and herpes)
- Medications (see chapter 5)
- Periods of vomiting and diarrhea

Chronic constipation

Chronic constipation can be caused by a variety of things, including laxative abuse (discussed in chapter 8); diseases affecting body tissues, nerve, or muscle control; inflammation, scarring, or blockage in the lower intestine; spinal injuries; prolonged bed rest or being bedridden (especially for seniors). Lack of exercise and poor diet are the most common causes of chronic constipation.

Hemorrhoids

The straining caused by chronic constipation can lead to hemorrhoids. These are swollen blood vessels or veins around the anus either inside (internal) or under the skin around it (external). A classic symptom of internal hemorrhoids is finding bright red blood covering your stool, on toilet paper, or in the toilet bowl. Sometimes an internal hemorrhoid protrudes through the rectum and hangs outside the body, known as a *protruding or prolapsing hemorrhoid*. Since bleeding is a problem with internal hemorrhoids, you can become anemic, but this is really unusual.

External hemorrhoids are characterized by swelling or a hard lump around the rectum (due to a blood clot). This is sometimes called a thrombosed external hemorrhoid (sounds terrible, but it isn't serious at all). It looks like an oversized blueberry. This will be irritating and painful. Straining, rubbing, or cleaning around the area will irritate it more, causing it to bleed or itch.

To find some relief, try warm tub or sitz baths (when the water just covers your "heinie") several times a day. Don't use anything in the water except a little baking soda (optional), and don't stay in longer than about ten minutes. Stool softeners may help you pass stool more comfortably, while ice packs will help reduce swelling (ten minutes on/ten minutes off). Frequently shifting positions while standing or sitting is helpful. Over-the-counter medication such as Preparation H can also give relief but won't shrink the hemorrhoid. If the problem is not resolving itself, the hemorrhoid can be removed in a doctor's office or through a minor surgical procedure in the hospital. Common surgical procedures include:

- **Rubber band ligation:** A rubber band placed around the base of an internal hemorrhoid, inside the rectum, cuts off circulation, causing the hemorrhoid to shrivel up.
- **Sclerotherapy:** A chemical solution is injected around the blood vessel to shrink an internal hemorrhoid.
- **Electrical or laser heat (laser coagulation) or infrared light (infrared photo coagulation):** These techniques are used to burn off external hemorrhoids.
- **Hemorrhoidectomy:** Surgical removal of an external hemorrhoid or severe internal hemorrhoid.

Diarrhea

Technically, diarrhea is defined as having liquid bowel movements for more than twelve hours. Most people have diarrhea from time to time. Temporary bouts of diarrhea are caused by an infection or food poisoning. Diarrhea is a problem when it's prolonged or chronic.

The infectious causes of diarrhea will tend to vary from region to region. There have been many reports about shigella, but the fact is, shigella is not the most common cause of infectious diarrhea. Viruses probably are. As for bacterial-related diarrhea, campylobacter jejuni, and salmonella (see further on) are probably more common than shigella.

Another common bacteria, *Clostridium difficile,* or *C. difficile,* grows when antibiotics kill off the bacteria that normally counteract *C. difficile*. This bacteria, discovered in the late 1970s, damages intestinal cells, causing diarrhea and colitis. These bacteria tend to flourish in hospitals because they can be harbored in bedpans, wheelchairs, linens, and so on, and on unwashed or ungloved hands. *C. difficile* is treated with vancomycin or metronidazole, as well as discontinuing the initial antibiotics which allowed *C. difficile* to develop.

There are numerous other food-borne illnesses, such as salmonella (raw eggs, undercooked chicken or ham), *E. coli* (undercooked red meat, such as hamburger), botulism (found in high-protein foods that are canned), staphylococcus (this isn't food-borne but gets into food from infected sores, pimples, and noses of food packers or handlers), as well as several parasites that can cause diarrhea. Unless your immune system is suppressed for some reason, these episodes usually pass—literally—with the aid of the BRAT diet (bananas, rice, applesauce, and tea) and an antidiarrheal medication such as Imodium.

Chronic diarrhea

If diarrhea is chronic, *and* is caused by an infection, follow the BRAT diet, drink fluids such as Gatorade to replace your electrolytes, and consider being tested for HIV. See chapter 8 for more details. Noninfectious, chronic diarrhea means you probably have a bowel disorder of some kind that requires further investigation, discussed in the next two sections.

IRRITABLE BOWELS?

A confusing label has come into vogue, which defines the bowel habits of between 25 and 55 million North Americans, two-thirds of whom are women. The label is *irritable bowel syndrome* (IBS), which refers to unusual bowel "patterns" that alternate between diarrhea and constipation, and everything in between. It tends to first strike people under the age of forty, often during their teen years. IBS affects Caucasians and African North Americans in equal numbers, but Hispanics suffer less IBS, a difference that may be related to diet. IBS is also referred to as irritable or spastic colon; spastic, mucus, nervous, laxative, cathartic, or functional colitis; spastic bowel; nervous indigestion; functional dyspepsia; pylorospasm; and functional bowel disease. The problem with using the term *irritable* is that irritation is *not* what's going on. It also sounds too much like "inflammatory," which is not what's going on either. Worse, many family doctors will say "IBS" instead of, "We don't know what's going on—but have you tried fiber?"

The term *irritable bowel syndrome* came into use to describe a bowel that is overly sensitive to normal activity. In other words, when the nerve endings that line the bowel are too sensitive, the nerves controlling the GI tract can become overactive, making the bowel overly responsive or "irritable" to normal things, such as passing gas or fluid. In other words, the bowel may want to pass a stool before it's time. The bowel, in a sense, becomes too "touchy" for comfort. However, since we tend to think of *irritable*, when the term is used clinically, as something that is red, irritated, or inflamed, this label is more confusing than defining. IBS has nothing to do with irritation, inflammation, or any organic disease process. It has to do with nerves.

The term IBS also implies that a diagnosis of symptoms has been made and there is a definite cause—and cure—for the condition. This is not so at all. IBS is a diagnosis made in the absence of any other diagnosis. There is no test to confirm IBS, only tests to rule out other causes for the symptoms. The term *functional bowel disorder* is beginning to catch on instead of IBS, because "functional" means there is no identifiable inflammation, growth, infection, and so on, and that the problem is one of abnormal function. But this doesn't mean that this is not a disease of the control of bowel motility. However, this term is about as descriptive as non-ulcer dyspepsia (discussed in chapter 4), because it tells you what is not rather than what is: It is not a disease that has an organic cause. In any event, neither term—IBS or functional bowel disorder—satisfactorily explains what's going on. Some doctors are beginning to use the term *unknown bowel disorder*, which is a little less deceptive. In clinical circles, IBS is categorized into a broader group of diseases known as functional gastrointestinal disorders, which includes non-ulcer dyspepsia, noncardiac chest pain, and chronic constipation or diarrhea. All of these disorders have one thing in common: no known biological or organic cause.

Yet no matter what you call it, roughly half of all digestive disorders are attributed to IBS. After the common cold, IBS is the chief cause of absenteeism. Many doctors compare IBS to asthma in that there are a number of causes with the same outcome. Asthma may be related to allergies or a hundred other things. Similarly, IBS has many different causes that are difficult to pin down. However, stress and dietary factors are the chief causes.

IBS Symptoms

IBS symptoms are characterized by frequent, violent episodes of diarrhea that almost always strike around a stressful situation. (People often experience IBS symptoms before job interviews or plane trips.) Over 60 percent of IBS sufferers report that their symptoms first coincided with stressful life events, while 40 to 60 percent of people with IBS also suffer from anxiety disorders or depression, compared to 20 percent of people with other GI disorders. Stressful life events that can bring on IBS include the death of a loved one, separation/divorce, unresolved conflict or grief, moving to a new city or job, as well as having a childhood history of physical or sexual abuse.

Many people find that their symptoms persist well beyond the stressful life event, and the episodes invade their normal routine. It need not be one, single stressful event that precipitates IBS; the condition could first present itself after you've been in a stressful job for a long time or been subjected to the normal stresses of "life in North America" for a long time. The episodes of diarrhea are often accompanied by crampy abdominal pains or gas, which are relieved by a bowel movement. The pain may shift around in the abdomen as well. After the diarrhea episodes, you may then be plagued by long bouts of constipation, or the feeling that you're not emptying your bowels completely when you do go. Again, IBS refers to an irregular bowel *pattern* rather than one particular episode. The pattern is that there is *no normal pattern* of bowel movements; it is often one extreme or the other.

Your stools may also contain mucus, which can make the stool long and ropelike or wormlike. The mucus is normally secreted by the colon to help the stool along in a normal movement. In IBS, the colon secretes too much mucus. However, blood mixed with the stools means this is not IBS, but something else. Some people can also suffer from diarrhea only, or gas and constipation only. Other symptoms include bloating, nausea, and loss of appetite. Fever, weight loss, or severe pain are *not* signs of IBS but of something else.

Many people find it confusing that IBS can cause both constipation and diarrhea, which seem to be opposite ends of the spectrum. But what happens is that instead of the slow muscular contractions that normally move the bowels, spasms occur, and these can either result in an "explosion" or a "blockage." It's akin to a sudden gust of wind; it can blow the door wide open (diarrhea), or blow it shut (constipation). It all depends on the direction of the wind.

It's important to note the timing of your diarrhea; in IBS, your sleep should not be disturbed by it. The episodes will always occur after a meal or in the early evening.

Factors that distinguish IBS from infectious diarrhea or inflammatory bowel diseases (see further on) are:

▣ finding relief through defecation
▣ noticing looser stools when the bowel movement is precipitated by pain
▣ noticing more frequent bowel movements when you experience pain
▣ noticing abdominal bloating or distention
▣ noticing mucus in the stools
▣ feeling that you have not completely emptied your bowels

What to Rule Out

The symptoms of IBS are a little vague in that they can be signs of many other GI problems. Therefore, before you accept a diagnosis of IBS, make sure your doctor has taken a careful history (see chapter 2) to investigate:

▣ dietary culprits, food allergies, lactose intolerance, or just plain "poor diet"—high fats/starch; low fiber
▣ intestinal bacterial, viral, or parasitic infections (where have you been traveling? what are your sexual habits?)
▣ overgrowth of *C. difficile* (see chapter 5)
▣ yeast in the GI tract (called candidiasis), which is notorious for causing IBS symptoms (eating yogurt every day should clear this up)
▣ medications (see chapter 5)
▣ stress (the GI tract, which is controlled by the nervous system, can definitely react when you're under stress)

▣ motility problems (discussed in chapter 4, many specialists believe that IBS is part of dysmotility)

▣ enzyme deficiencies (the pancreas may not be secreting enough enzymes to break down food)

▣ serious disease such as inflammatory bowel disease (see further on) or signs of cancer

Your doctor can rule out all the above by requesting a stool sample to check for blood or infections, and a culture for bacteria or parasite eggs (several stool samples over the course of a month are recommended). Endoscopy will rule out serious bowel diseases such as ulcerative colitis or Crohn's disease (see below), while a few general blood tests over the course of a month can also help to rule out various infections.

Recent studies show that people who have suffered from food poisoning are prone to IBS symptoms thereafter, suggesting that somehow the infection has either not passed through completely or has altered bowel function. In one study, one in four people with bacterial infections in their intestinal tract later reported IBS symptoms.

Treating IBS

Once other causes for symptoms have been ruled out, the only treatment is to pay close attention to diet, as well as taking over-the-counter or herbal antidiarrheals or laxatives. That means keeping a diary to chart which foods seem to trigger episodes, as well as adopting a low-fat, high-fiber diet (which is discussed at length in chapter 9). Fat, for example, stimulates the colon to contract after eating. Diets low in sugar are also recommended. In fact, some over-the-counter fiber preparations are so loaded with sugar that they may not be of any benefit.

Avoiding foods high in lectins, such as tomatoes and

strawberries, may also help to prevent diarrhea. If you're having an episode of diarrhea, the BRAT diet—bananas, rice, applesauce, and tea—is the one to follow. Studies also show that certain antihistamines can counteract diarrhea.

A word about stress

It's possible to have a pristine diet, rule out all forms of organic disease, yet still suffer from IBS while under stress. In the same way that you can sweat, blush, or cry under emotional stress, your GI tract may also react to stress by "weeping"—producing excessive water and mucus, overreacting to normal stimuli such as eating. What often happens, however, is that there is a delayed "gut reaction" to stress, and you may not experience IBS symptoms until the stress has passed. Apparently, under stress your brain becomes more active as a defense. (For example, when we're running away from a predator, we have to think quickly and act quickly, so our heart rate increases, we sweat more, and so on.) During this "defensive mode" the entire nervous system can become exaggerated (that's what causes "butterflies in the stomach"). The nerves controlling the GI tract therefore become highly sensitive, causing IBS symptoms. Studies show, for example, that IBS symptoms are more common on weekday mornings than on afternoons or weekends, while IBS symptoms do not appear at night during sleep.

If you find that your stress is unmanageable, it's probably time to seek some help through a counselor, therapist, or support group. Many people find that their IBS symptoms dissipate after they get their lives back in order.

Women and IBS

Why is IBS more common in women? For one thing, women menstruate and experience normal mood fluctuations related to their natural menstrual cycles. Mood changes are common premenstrual symptoms that may create more emotional stress, and hence IBS symptoms. Another factor is uterine contractions during menstruation. When the uterus contracts, it often stimulates a bowel movement. The first day of a woman's period is often a day where she has several loose bowel movements. Meanwhile, common symptoms of labor include diarrhea and vomiting. These occur because of the intensity of the uterine contractions, which create "ripples" throughout the GI tract.

Women who experience painful periods or endometriosis may also experience IBS symptoms more intensely. In endometriosis, parts of the uterine lining grow outside the uterus, into the abdominal cavity, often triggering painful bowel movements, diarrhea, or constipation during or just prior to menstruation. For more information on endometriosis, consult my book *The Gynecological Sourcebook*.

Finally, women are much more prone to eating disorders and laxative abuse, as well as domestic abuse (resulting in continuous emotional upset and stress), all of which wreak havoc on the gastrointestinal tract. This is discussed in more detail in chapter 8.

INFLAMMATORY REMARKS

There is a huge difference between irritable bowel syndrome and inflammatory bowel disease (IBD). The latter is a serious, chronic condition that can be life-threatening in extreme cases. IBD means that one or more parts of the small or large intestine are inflamed, causing symptoms that range from unpleasant but manageable to severe and debilitating.

When inflammation and/or ulceration is confined to the inner lining of the colon (colitis) and rectum (proctitis), you have what's known as ulcerative colitis. The inflammation will usually start in the rectum and then spread throughout the colon. Because it's inflamed, the colon will not be able to do what it was designed to do: hold solid waste. As a result, it will need to empty waste as soon as it receives it; you'll experience this as diarrhea. The inflammation will cause the cells that line the colon to slough off or die, which may cause open sores on the lining (ulcers), which could then form pus or mucus. So the diarrhea is often tinged with blood, pus, or mucus.

When the inflammation goes beyond the lining into the actual walls of the intestine, you have what's known as Crohn's disease, which usually attacks north of the colon, in the ileum. For this reason, Crohn's disease is also known as ileitis or regional enteritis. Crohn's disease can also attack the colon or other parts of the GI tract.

If the intestines were a trench coat, ulcerative colitis would be confined to the lining of the coat below the belt; Crohn's disease would affect the entire coat starting at the belt, possibly all the way up to the collar. Or it could start at the belt and affect everything below it.

Who Gets IBD?

North America is a "hotbed" for IBD, affecting both men and women of all ages and races. IBD seems to flare up in people aged fifteen to thirty-five or in people over fifty. It is believed to be an autoimmune disorder, where the immune system attacks its own body tissues. Autoimmune diseases tend to be inherited and are more common in people who already have other autoimmune diseases. Roughly 20 percent of all people with IBD have family members with IBD. Other autoimmune diseases include lupus, multiple sclerosis, various thyroid diseases, and rheumatoid arthritis.

Some studies show that an intestinal bacteria seems to be at work, too, which somehow causes the autoimmune response in people who have inherited IBD genes. (This is a similar idea to the "*H. pylori* story" in chapter 3.) For example, it's known that bacteria can stimulate the production of proteins called cytokines that cause inflammation. If a specific bacteria is identified, then it could perhaps be destroyed before it does any damage. Researchers are also trying to find ways to stop the inflammatory response before it starts, as well as to identify specific IBD genes. Other studies are looking into a cattle bacteria (related to tuberculosis) known as *Mycobacterium paratuberculosis* as a possible cause of Crohn's disease, which may explain why it's most common in regions that consume a lot of beef, such as North America, England, and northern Europe. Ulcerative colitis, in particular, is much more common in Jewish people, and is rare in Asian and black people. But as underdeveloped countries become more Westernized, IBD is seen more often.

Smoking or nonsmoking?

Ulcerative colitis is not only more prevalent among nonsmokers or ex-smokers, it is even said to be a "disease of nonsmokers." No one knows why this is, but studies that have used nicotine skin patches as a drug therapy for ulcerative colitis show that people actually improve when other drugs have not been successful. Nevertheless, smokers still develop high rates of lung cancer and cardiovascular problems. Crohn's disease, on the other hand, is much more common in smokers than in nonsmokers.

In a recent Mayo Clinic study, the use of high-dose nicotine skin patches significantly helped control the symptoms of ulcerative colitis in nearly 40 percent of colitis patients studied. Other studies using lower doses of nicotine did not find that symptoms improved; it's thought that the high-dose nicotine patch is the only effective nicotine therapy. But high-dose nicotine patches can cause side effects such as skin rashes, nausea, and dizziness.

Symptoms of Ulcerative Colitis

Abdominal cramps combined with bloody diarrhea (which could contain mucus and/or pus) and frequent, *urgent* bowel movements are the most common signs of ulcerative colitis. The diarrhea usually strikes immediately after meals or at night. Some people may also lose control of their bowel movements (called fecal incontinence) or pass stool in the belief that it is just gas. Obviously, these symptoms can interfere with many daily activities, including sleeping. Not all people will suffer from severe symptoms. It depends on where the inflammation is. Sometimes it's confined to the rectum or to one side of the colon versus the entire colon.

When symptoms are severe, you can suffer from all of the following:

- fatigue
- weight loss
- loss of appetite and/or nausea
- rectal bleeding
- malnutrition (mainly due to the loss of fluids and nutrients)
- anemia (from bleeding)

The same causes that trigger the immune system to attack the bowel tissue can also cause it to attack other body tissues, causing complications such as skin lesions, arthritis, inflammation of the eyes, or liver disorders, including jaundice and cirrhosis, which could necessitate a liver transplant.

In severe but rare cases, known as toxic megacolon, the colon enlarges and distends. This will cause fever, abdominal pain, dehydration, and malnutrition. In this case, surgery is necessary to prevent the colon from rupturing.

Symptoms of Crohn's Disease

The symptoms of Crohn's disease are similar to those of ulcerative colitis: abdominal cramps and diarrhea, resulting in rectal bleeding, anemia, weight loss, and fever (fever is not usually a symptom in ulcerative colitis unless the colon enlarges). The fever may make it easy for Crohn's disease to be confused with infectious diarrhea. The location of the abdominal cramping in Crohn's disease is usually in the lower right side.

Because Crohn's disease attacks the intestinal walls and can occur higher up in the GI tract, obstruction can take place due to narrowing of passageways (they swell and develop scar tissue). Fistulas ("ulcer tunnels" between tissues) can develop around the bladder, rectum, anus, or vagina. These tunnels can become infected and filled with pus. They are a common complication and often are associated with pockets of infection or abscesses (infected areas of pus).

As in ulcerative colitis, the autoimmune nature of Crohn's disease can also cause other body parts to inflame, including joints, skin, eyes, and mouth. Kidney stones and gallstones (see chapter 7) are other complications related to Crohn's disease.

Ulcerative Colitis or Crohn's?

Since the symptoms of ulcerative colitis and Crohn's disease are virtually indistinguishable, the only way to tell which disease the patient has is to examine the bowel tissue under a microscope. This is done by a pathologist (a doctor who specializes in analyzing tissue specimens under a microscope). Some pathologists specialize in gastroenterology. A gastroenterologist can get a tissue sample through a procedure known as sigmoidoscopy (where a short tube with a lighted microscope on the end is inserted through the rectum) or colonoscopy (where a similar but much longer tube is inserted while you're under sedation via intravenous).

Your doctor will also want to collect a stool sample to rule out infections or parasites, which can also cause mucus or pus-tinged diarrhea. Finally, blood tests will confirm whether you're anemic or have a high white blood cell count, a sign of inflammation. In some cases, a barium enema (a chalky solution inserted into the colon, which shows up on X-ray film) can also help to confirm where inflammation is.

If Crohn's disease is suspected, you'll probably have an upper GI series (see chapter 2) as well, which can reveal whether there is any inflammation in the upper GI tract.

Taking a thorough history (see chapter 2) is also important when trying to pin down IBD. Your family history is crucial, since IBD tends to run in families, while a family history of colorectal cancer is also a sign that ulcerative colitis, in particular, runs in the family. (Cancer risk is discussed further on.)

Both ulcerative colitis and Crohn's disease can last a lifetime or a few months. Many people experience long bouts of symptom-free living (months or years), but IBD has a tendency to recur and is considered a chronic disease.

Treating IBD

Treating IBD depends on where the inflammation is and how severe symptoms are. In mild ulcerative colitis, for example (where inflammation is limited to the rectum or end of the left colon), treatments can be as simple as oral medications or an occasional enema. There are usually "trigger foods" such as dairy products or spicy food, and avoiding these can help prevent flare-ups in mild IBD.

For people with severe IBD, strong medications are necessary, discussed separately below under "IBD Drugs."

When complications from the disease set in, the patient may need to be hospitalized to replenish nutrients or body fluids through intravenous feeding. Often the treatment for IBD is "palliative" in that treatment focuses on the "symptoms of the week"; in the case of Crohn's disease, this is about all that can be done.

When Surgery Is Necessary

Surgery can cure ulcerative colitis, but not Crohn's disease (although it may help). In the first case, since the inflammation is confined to the colon and rectum, removal of the colon and rectum removes the problem. However, since Crohn's disease travels all over the GI tract, and can recur, surgery isn't considered a "cure-all."

Removing the colon (colectomy)

Roughly one-quarter of all people with ulcerative colitis will need to have their colons surgically removed due to severe bleeding, chronic illness, or perforation of the colon. This is usually a last resort when drug therapy fails.

The surgery used to treat ulcerative colitis is called a procto-colectomy, where the entire colon and rectum are removed, and the tip of the ileum (the lower small intestine) is pulled down and out of a neat, quarter-sized hole (called a stoma) made through the abdominal wall around the belt line. An external pouch, called an ostomy device, is placed over the ileum's tip to allow waste to drain out; the patient removes and replaces the pouch when it's full (similar to changing a vacuum cleaner bag). This entire procedure is known as an ileostomy. This operation allows for continence, but does not result in a normal bowel movement. At best, people who undergo this procedure have four to six bowel movements per day and may have some leakage—especially at night. A newer procedure, called a continent ileostomy, creates a waste pouch inside the intestinal wall, which acts as a "dummy rectum."

There are variations of this operation where the rectum is saved, not requiring the wearing of a pouch. In this case, the colon is removed and the ileum is "pulled down" and surgically attached to the rectum, allowing normal defecation (bowel movements will be watery and more frequent, however). If the rectum is in bad shape, another procedure can rebuild the rectum using the ileum. The new rectum is then stitched to the anus, also allowing normal defecation. This is akin to cutting off a section of a garden hose and then sewing the two ends together. The pouch operation is the favored procedure, however.

Some things to keep in mind

About 100,000 ostomy surgeries are performed annually, while at least one million North Americans have ostomy devices. The surgery itself is quite simple, although it obviously changes one's life. A few men become impotent following ostomy surgery, but most men are fully able to have an erection and orgasm after the surgery.

Women will also be fully able to become pregnant without any impaired sexual function. Only in a few cases, where complications occur within the abdominal cavity, does ostomy surgery necessitate a hysterectomy.

Repair surgery

This kind of surgery is reserved for severe cases of Crohn's disease where parts of the intestine have narrowed (called a stricture) or become blocked, perforated, or abscessed. Surgery is used to drain abscesses or remove various blocks (known as a surgical resection). The problem is that too many resection surgeries can lead to a situation where there simply is not enough of the bowel left to absorb any nutrients; this is known as short-bowel or "short gut" syndrome. To avoid this problem, innovations in Crohn's surgery have yielded a newer procedure known as strictureplasty, where the stricture is widened without removing any part of the bowel.

If you currently have short-bowel syndrome, intestinal transplants can be performed but are still in the experimental stage and are not widely available. However, studies to date show that Crohn's disease can recur in a transplanted bowel within seven months of the transplant.

IBD Drugs

Over-the-counter medications that can relieve symptoms of IBS are not appropriate in IBD. That's because the problem is inflammation caused by an autoimmune disease. Drugs that control inflammation or suppress the immune system are therefore the first choice in treating either ulcerative colitis or Crohn's disease. All the drugs discussed in this section are very powerful, have side effects, and must never be combined with any other drug without consulting your doctor and pharmacist.

The salicylates

The salicylates are a group of drugs that can reduce inflammation, especially in the colon. Examples of salicylate drugs include sufasalazine, olsalazine, and mesalamine. These drugs are considered a good start because they can be taken in high doses, can be combined with other drugs, and are usually well-tolerated. That said, not everyone will do well on salicylates. Side effects include nausea, vomiting, weight loss, heartburn, and more diarrhea.

Corticosteroids

The next step is a more powerful steroid drug, such as prednisone or hydrocortisone, which controls inflammation and suppresses the immune system. Corticosteroids were discovered in the 1950s. These drugs mimic cortisol, an anti-inflammatory hormone made by the adrenal gland. (The late John F. Kennedy used very high doses of this drug to help relieve symptoms from severe back problems, complicated by Addison's disease, a disease of the adrenal gland.) The problem with steroid drugs is that they carry some serious long-term side effects. People who have used steroid drugs for long periods of time can be vulnerable to bone thinning, muscle deterioration, and various skin problems, including a puffy face. Infections, pancreatic damage, and some neurological problems can also develop. But you can't go off steroid drugs when you feel like it, because stopping the medication suddenly can cause withdrawal symptoms, which can include weakness, fatigue, menstrual cycle changes in women, decreased appetite, weight loss, nausea, vomiting, and diarrhea (again!). Many of these symptoms can be confused with a recurrence of IBD. To prevent withdrawal symptoms, steroid drug dosages are gradually decreased.

Immunosuppressants

If inflammation is still not controlled, there are more powerful immunosuppressant drugs (also known as immune modulator drugs) often used in cancer therapy, such as azathioprine or 6-mercaptopurine. Since IBD is thought to be an autoimmune disease, suppressing the immune system has been shown to help "call off the attack" on intestinal tissues. These drugs can also help you to gradually go off steroid drugs, which will minimize any long-term side effects. Cyclosporine and methotrexate, other common anticancer drugs, are also used in extreme cases of IBD.

These medications are also used frequently in transplant patients to prevent tissue rejection. The problem with these drugs is that they don't offer immediate benefits; it takes several months for them to take effect, which means that side effects can set in before any benefits do.

Cytokine blockers

These are the newest class of drugs added to IBD therapy. Researchers have discovered that cytokines are produced during inflammation. These are proteins that cause inflammation. Drugs aimed specifically at these cytokines are a promising new trend in IBD therapy, but are not yet available unless you are in a specific research trial.

DIVERTICULOSIS

An extremely common condition among adults over sixty is the development of small, pea-sized sacs in the wall of the colon, known as diverticulosis. (The sacs are called diverticuli.) They form in areas where the colon is weakened, due to a history of bowel diseases or often simply aging.

The majority of North Americans probably have diverticulosis but don't realize it. These sacs generally don't cause any symptoms unless they become inflamed for some reason (known as diverticulitis), which can cause bleeding or tearing in about 20 percent of the cases.

The Symptoms

Usually there are no symptoms, but when there are, you may feel some tenderness or muscle spasms in one area of the abdomen. The lower left side of the abdomen may feel painful and tender. Occasionally the pain can be in the middle or on the right side.

When inflammation occurs, you'll definitely have symptoms, such as fever, a high white blood cell count, and abdominal pain.

If the sacs become infected, they may bleed or form pus, which can block your bowel or cause the bowel wall to break (known as a perforation). This is an emergency situation that requires immediate surgery.

SCREENING FOR COLON CANCER

Anyone over the age of forty-five is at risk for colorectal (colon and/or rectal) cancer. The risk is about thirty-two times higher if you have ulcerative colitis for at least ten years. That's because ulcerative colitis can cause the cells that line the colon to become precancerous (known as dysplasia). If only the rectum or lower part of the colon is involved, the risk is no higher than in the general population.

Nevertheless, if you've had ulcerative colitis for more than eight years, you should be screened every two years for evidence of dysplasia through endoscopy (sigmoidoscopy or colonoscopy) and biopsies. If dysplasia is found, you may be offered the option of a colectomy to prevent the spread of precancerous cells and the development of full-blown colon cancer.

Screening in the General Population

In the general population, one in twenty people with no known risk factors for colorectal cancer will develop it. Anytime you experience what's defined in chapter 2 as an "alarm symptom," you should definitely see your doctor to investigate the problem. These symptoms include changes in bowel habits, stool consistency, blood in the stools, and so on. You should also have an annual occult blood test (a test checking for "hidden" blood in the stools) as part of your annual physical exam. Having an annual rectal exam is also recommended after age forty-five.

Known risk factors for colorectal cancer include a history of ulcerative colitis, a family history of colorectal, breast, or ovarian cancers, a history of benign tumors in the colon or rectum (called polyps), and a diet high in fat and low in fiber.

If you are concerned about your risk and are over forty-five, you should request a workup that includes a flexible sigmoidoscopy, a colonoscopy, barium enema, and a full blood workup. If you're all clear, then a workup every five years is appropriate thereafter. Chapter 9 discusses in more detail the "Recipe for Prevention" regarding colon cancer.

The abdominal pains that accompany many of the bowel problems discussed in this chapter can also have other sources. Because your GI tract is a "high traffic" area for many other organs, traffic jams can occur, causing more symptoms and discomfort.

CHAPTER 7

THE TROUBLE WITH ABS

While your lungs may have a lot of "breathing room," your intestines are crammed into a ghetto with your liver, gallbladder, appendix, and pancreas. While these organs perform separate operations, they all work in the same industry: digestion and food distribution. When all your organs are working properly, you don't even notice how close the quarters are. However, when one of these "houses" is not in order, you'll feel it in the form of GI symptoms. This chapter is an overview of the GI neighborhood so that you have a better idea of what's inside your abdominal cavity, what can go wrong, and which symptoms warrant immediate medical attention.

WEST SIDE STORY

If you imagine your digestive tract (mouth, esophagus, stomach, and small and large intestines) as a river that flows north to south, your liver, gallbladder, and appendix are situated on the riverbanks to the west. To the east is the pancreas. The liver and pancreas make digestive juices that get sent, through various ducts, into the duodenum. The gallbladder acts as an extra storage tank for the liver, and the appendix is nothing more than a "museum piece" left over from primitive humans.

The Mighty Liver

If the kidneys are the "public servants" of the body (controlling hydro and garbage pickup), the liver is the giant recycling plant, where everything your body ingests is carefully sorted, and usually recycled, with the exception of poisonous or hazardous wastes (such as those found in various medications), which are sent to the large intestine for elimination. The liver is large; it weighs in at around four pounds, and you have much more of it than you really need to live. In fact, the liver can function when 50 percent of it is destroyed; unlike the kidneys, however, you only have one liver.

The liver makes bile, which is crucial for breaking down fat, which is absorbed into the cells through the intestines. After the intestines absorb the nutrients they want, the liver revisits the unabsorbed molecules, such as amino acids and sugars, and "makes some calls" to other parts of the body to see if these molecules can be used. Usually they are used. Whatever is left over is stored by the liver for later use. For example, it's usually left with lots of extra glucose, which it doesn't have room to store. Therefore, the liver converts the glucose into glycogen, which can be reconverted into sugar at a moment's notice. (Glycogen is a key player in diabetes.) The liver doesn't store that much fat, although fat can accumulate in the liver in certain diseases. What the liver does do is make fat particles (from fatty acids and glycerol), which are then transported through the bloodstream to other tissues. The liver also manufactures cholesterol, which the body needs in normal amounts. This is the one substance that is not stored by the liver for future use. The liver makes cholesterol from the fats it receives and sends it out into the bloodstream. If you eat too much of certain fats (tropical oils are the worst), the liver manufactures cholesterol. If you ingest a food that is naturally high in cholesterol—such as liver or egg yolks—the cholesterol will simply stay in your body. Too much cholesterol is a bad thing and will clog your blood vessels.

All the vitamins, minerals, and medications you ingest get sent to the liver, too. The liver is able to store excess vitamins, distribute necessary vitamins to the cells that need them, as well as remove many of the toxins that come into the body in the form of environmental toxins, medications, and so on. People who regularly take strong medications or abuse drugs or alcohol put a strain on the liver—which is designed to handle some abuse, but not too much.

When the liver catches a virus

The liver is vulnerable to three kinds of viral infections: hepatitis A, hepatitis B, and hepatitis C. (Actually, there are a few more versions of hepatitis, but there are no blood tests yet to confirm them.) Hepatitis means inflammation of the liver. No matter which version of hepatitis you're infected with, the symptoms are the same, but can take up to 180 days to manifest. The first phase of hepatitis symptoms is the worst. You may experience diarrhea, vomiting, fever, nausea, and sometimes skin lesions or joint inflammation. The second phase can cause flulike symptoms, jaundice (yellowing of the skin, because the liver is not reusing red blood cells properly), darker urine, and lighter stools (due to a reduction in bile).

Some forms of hepatitis do not cause any symptoms but will damage the liver nonetheless. Most people recover from hepatitis but may remain weak for some time.

The most important aspect about hepatitis is that it can be prevented. Hepatitis B is transmitted through blood or bodily fluids, and is therefore a sexually transmitted disease like HIV. Safe sex and safe needle use will prevent hepatitis B. There is also a vaccine for hepatitis B. Hepatitis A is passed on like staphylococcus (see chapter 6), through an infected food handler who passes the virus through contaminated food or water. There is, fortunately, a vaccine to prevent hepatitis A. There is no vaccine yet for hepatitis C, which can be passed on through blood transfusions, although it is specifically screened for in blood.

Cirrhosis of the liver

Cirrhosis is a condition where the liver becomes scarred by infections, such as hepatitis, or by toxic chemicals. In the Western world, 75 percent of all cases of cirrhosis are caused by alcoholism. However, in underdeveloped parts of the world, hepatitis is the major cause of cirrhosis. Cirrhosis is also seen in children, where it is frequently caused by cystic fibrosis or other inherited disorders. Whenever you see the phrase "liver toxicity" as a risk factor from various medications, this refers to liver damage *not* specifically due to cirrhosis, also known as "drug-induced liver toxicity." When a drug enters your bloodstream, your liver converts it into usable chemicals, removing toxins the body cannot use or tolerate. However, in the same way that a worker can be exposed to toxic fumes if it is his job to clean them up, the liver becomes exposed. The more toxins the liver removes, the more damage it incurs. When drugs are damaging your liver, you will experience the following symptoms:

- severe fatigue
- abdominal pain and swelling
- jaundice (yellow eyes and skin, dark urine)
- fever
- nausea or vomiting

The only way to tell whether these symptoms are drug-induced or viral-related is to stop your medications to see if you get better.

Large amounts of acetaminophen (especially when combined with alcohol), anticonvulsants, antihypertensive methyldopa, chlorpromazine, drugs used to treat tuberculosis, and too much vitamin A or niacin are classic causes of drug-induced liver damage. Acetaminophen taken as prescribed, however, will not cause liver damage.

Liver toxicity can also occur from exposure to environmental toxins, such as benzene (common in many cleaning fluids).

Treating cirrhosis

There is no way to treat cirrhosis of the liver; it is a serious, debilitating condition in which the liver eventually stops working. When the cirrhosis is caused by a known toxin or alcohol, if the toxin is removed, the liver sometimes recovers enough to function (it can rebuild itself). But one of the problems with treating liver disease is that no medications can be used, since they must be metabolized in the liver. The only choice you have when your liver ceases to function is to have a liver transplant, which is not available to most people. The word *live* is in *liver* for a reason: You can't live without it. When it breaks down, you break down.

The Gallbladder

As discussed above, the gallbladder stores bile for the liver. But you don't really need the gallbladder, since the liver is large enough to store as much bile as you'd ever need. Nevertheless, we come equipped with this extra storage space. Bile isn't a very reliable product to store because it can form little stones inside the gallbladder, known as gallstones or calculi. Roughly 10 percent of the North American population has gallstones. Many don't realize it because there may be no symptoms. Symptoms occur when the stones become large enough to obstruct the bile ducts. When this happens, you are said to have gallbladder disease.

The symptoms are quite severe: sudden, intense pain in the upper abdominal region (which may shoot into your back), often after a fatty meal, but often not related to meals. Vomiting often brings relief, although nausea is not a symptom. The pain may then subside over several minutes or hours. Many people mistake gallstone symptoms for heartburn or a heart attack.

The obstruction can become infected, and even develop gangrene, which is a dire emergency (you don't want gangrene inside your abdominal cavity!). Usually gallbladder disease presents itself as a series of gallbladder attacks where you'll feel pain after a meal; if there's infection, you may have a fever. The attacks will become progressively worse until you decide to have the darned thing removed. As a rule, any abdominal pain accompanied by fever means there is some sort of serious infection, which warrants emergency medical attention.

Who will develop gallstones?

Gallstones are caused by a variety of things, including body chemistry, weight, diet, and how frequently the gallbladder empties. Many gallstones, for example, contain too much cholesterol and not enough bile salts, which can cause the cholesterol to crystallize and turn into a stone. There are also various proteins in the liver and bile that can either prevent cholesterol from crystallizing or cause it to crystallize.

As for body weight, studies show that obesity is a definite risk factor for gallstones; it's believed that the factors that cause weight gain may also influence the cholesterol content of the bile. It is the cholesterol levels in bile, rather than the blood cholesterol levels, that predisposes a person to gallstones. The factors that increase the risk of stones either increase cholesterol in bile or reduce the acid concentrations in bile. Meanwhile, the more cholesterol in the bile, the more slowly the gallbladder empties, giving the cholesterol more of an opportunity to crystallize.

On the other side of the coin, people who fast for long periods of time or go on very low calorie diets also develop gallstones, not because they have high cholesterol but because, it is presumed, they lose too much bile salt. The weight-gallbladder story is still not considered conclusive, but researchers have noted that low-fiber, high-cholesterol diets and diets high in starchy foods may contribute to gallstones.

We do know that an increase in estrogen will definitely increase cholesterol levels in bile. Gallbladder problems are therefore much more common in women than in men (one in five women after age fifty versus one in twenty men). They are also common during or after pregnancy, and in women who are on hormone replacement therapy after menopause. Estrogen-containing oral contraceptives are also associated with gallstones.

Since the late 1980s, gastroenterologists have been able to widen the bile ducts with endoscopy to remove stones in the bile duct, but this does not allow for the removal of stones in the gallbladder. In other words, it is used in a special situation and is not an alternative to gallbladder surgery.

When you need gallbladder surgery

The gallbladder is never taken out unless the patient is experiencing gallstones. Surgery to remove the gallbladder is invasive, even though the use of laparoscopy makes the surgery far less invasive than it used to be. Removal of the gallbladder is called a cholecystectomy, one of the most common surgical procedures performed. Over half a million North Americans have their gallbladder removed annually.

In the past, a cholecystectomy was major abdominal surgery, where a hole five to eight inches wide was made in the abdomen through which the gallbladder was removed. This required about a weeklong hospital stay and several weeks of recovery at home. Today, most cholecystectomies are done through laparoscopy, where several small incisions are made in the abdomen. With the aid of a video camera and a small instrument with a telescope on its end, the organs and tissues are magnified and a surgeon can easily separate the gallbladder from the liver and remove it without cutting any abdominal muscles. This translates into much less pain, faster healing, and a much lower risk of infection developing around the scar line. After laparoscopic surgery, you'll only need to stay overnight in the hospital and can recover for the next week at home.

A laparoscopic cholecystectomy still carries some complications, however. If the common bile duct is damaged during surgery, it can lead to a dangerous infection that may require corrective surgery. And in about 5 percent of all cholecystectomies, adhesions in the abdominal region can block the surgeon's view and necessitate the standard procedure, which is major surgery.

The Appendix

The appendix (clinically known as the veriform, or "wormlike" appendix) is attached to a section of the colon, and is believed to have played a role in primitive humans in digesting vegetation (such as tree bark or leaves). Who knows? Perhaps if you were stranded in Jurassic Park and started eating tree bark, your body might use the appendix again. But for now, the appendix serves no known biological purpose. The only reason I mention it is because it has a bad habit of becoming infected, inflamed, and then bursting into the abdominal cavity, causing the membrane lining the abdominal cavity (the peritoneum) to inflame, a condition known as peritonitis. Peritonitis is a very painful and life-threatening situation.

Appendicitis (inflammation of the appendix)

It's worth noting that prior to the late nineteenth century, people did not seem to suffer from appendicitis at all, leading some experts to believe that a change in diet over the last century has something to do with the cause of appendicitis. Just one attack warrants having the appendix surgically removed. The symptoms of appendicitis are two kinds of abdominal pain: (1) severe abdominal pain on the lower right side; (2) a general feeling of abdominal discomfort, resembling gas pains. Diarrhea or a continuous urge to defecate, as well as nausea, vomiting, a loss of appetite, and fever are all common symptoms. The symptoms usually develop during a period of six to eighteen hours. If you experience sharp pain on the lower right side, fever of over 101 degrees Fahrenheit, and pain when you move your abdomen or cough or sneeze, it's a sign of rupture. This is an emergency warranting an immediate appendectomy.

THE LOWER EAST SIDE

In New York City's lower East Side, many of the residents work two jobs to make ends meet. The pancreas, a bird beak–shaped gland behind the duodenum, pointing east, is no different. You might say it, too, leads a double life. It functions as both an exocrine gland (called the exocrine pancreas) as well as an endocrine gland (called the endocrine pancreas). The exocrine pancreas produces pancreatic enzymes that are released into the duodenum to digest food. These enzymes include amylase and lipase, which help to break down sugars and fats. The endocrine pancreas produces insulin, which is a hormone that regulates blood sugar levels, as well as glucagon (which is what signals your liver to convert glycogen into glucose).

Pancreatitis

When the bile ducts become blocked (perhaps by gallstones), bile can leak into the pancreas, triggering the enzymes to digest something—except the only thing in the pancreas to digest is the pancreas itself. As it's attacked by its own enzymes, it becomes inflamed, which is known as pancreatitis. This can lead to bleeding, tissue damage, cysts, and even diabetes if the insulin-producing cells are damaged. The result of pancreatitis is a big mess, as enzymes and toxins enter the bloodstream and damage other organs.

About a third of all cases of pancreatitis are caused by alcoholism. The rest of the cases are largely due to gallstones, but about 15 percent of the time the cause is unknown. Acute pancreatitis is a sudden flare-up that usually resolves itself after treatment.

In an acute case, the symptoms are quite severe. Constant abdominal pain will travel into the back or through the shoulders. Eating will make the pain worse, and the abdomen will feel swollen and tender. Nausea, vomiting, fever, and an increased pulse rate may accompany this pain, and the patient feels and looks quite sick. Dehydration and low blood pressure happen roughly 20 percent of the time, when the kidneys are affected. In short, this is a very critical infection.

During an attack, high levels of amylase will be found in the blood, including abnormal levels of calcium, magnesium, sodium, potassium, and bicarbonate. If the insulin-producing cells are affected, high blood sugar and cholesterol levels may also be high. Pancreatitis will get better on its own—and it's a good thing, since there really is no known treatment for acute pancreatitis, although there are ways to control the damage to other organs.

For example, intravenous fluids may be required to restore body chemistry or prevent other organs from failing. Antibiotics can also help to control infection, and sometimes surgery is needed to remove cysts, control bleeding, repair the bile duct, or remove the gallbladder. Incredibly, the pancreas recovers and the patient can usually carry on as before.

Chronic pancreatitis

Chronic pancreatitis rarely develops in people who are not alcoholics; 90 percent of all chronic pancreatitis is caused by alcoholism. The symptoms of chronic pancreatitis are identical to the acute attacks described above. However, in chronic pancreatitis, by the time an attack occurs, too much damage has been done. Chronic pancreatitis is more common in men than in women and is not seen before age thirty. Eventually, chronic pancreatitis, aside from the pain, leads to insulin-dependent diabetes. Fortunately, this can be treated with insulin and diet, while the pancreatic enzymes can be taken orally. In extreme cases, the pancreas is removed altogether. If you suffer from chronic pancreatitis, you *must* stop drinking, in addition to taking insulin and pancreatic enzymes orally.

HIS AND HERNIAS

Has your big toe ever broken through your sock? Well, essentially, that's what a hernia is: an organ that protrudes through its own cavity wall. The GI hernias are hiatal hernia and inguinal hernia. A hiatal hernia is when a portion of the stomach pokes out into the natural gap (*hiatus* means "gap") between the diaphragm and esophagus, which separates the respiratory system from the digestive tract. This is much more common in women than in men because it can be caused by pregnancy.

An inguinal hernia (a groin hernia) is when a portion of the intestinal tract pokes through the groin. Women get these, too, but because the testicles and scrotum have less support than the ligaments supporting the ovaries, men are more prone to inguinal hernias than are women.

Symptoms of Hiatal Hernia

When you have a hiatal hernia, stomach acid gets into the opening, causing symptoms of heartburn and reflux. Actually, the symptoms of hiatus hernia are those of GERD since that is what really is going on. The hiatus hernia is just one other factor contributing to GERD. Surgery is used when there is severe GERD that is not controlled by medication. It can be brought on by coughing, vomiting, straining while defecating, or sudden physical exertion. Pregnancy can cause the condition, as well as obesity, but aging is also a factor. Many people over fifty have small hiatal hernias. Unless you suffer from severe GERD or esophagitis (see chapter 4), which can complicate a hiatal hernia, you may not require any treatment. If the hernia does cause symptoms, surgery can repair it.

Symptoms of Inguinal Hernias

In this case, the only symptoms are feeling a lump in the scrotum, which may make you think it's a tumor instead of part of your lower intestines. When you lie down, the lump will go away as the abdomen flattens. If you feel any pain, it's a sign that the hernia has strangulated, cutting off blood flow to the intestines. In this case you'll feel pain and swelling because infection will set in. The treatment is an outpatient emergency repair surgery.

Almost without exception, each of the organs discussed in this chapter can get infected and inflamed and somehow cause peritonitis, inflammation of the abdominal wall. Anytime you experience abdominal pain and fever (with or without other symptoms, such as diarrhea or nausea), get yourself to a hospital emergency room for evaluation. Abdominal pain plus fever equals MAJOR INFECTION. It could be anything, but it's usually not "nothing." That's the only rule you should remember. Trying to decipher which side your pain is on, or what kind of pain it is (diffuse, acute, severe, "really bad," etc.) is a waste of time. The fever tells all. If you experience abdominal pain with other symptoms that do not include fever, this is not an emergency, but definitely warrants a visit to your doctor to find the source of the pain. The next chapter is devoted to people in special circumstances, who may suffer GI problems due to other diseases, such as AIDS, diabetes, anorexia or bulimia nervosa, endometriosis, and dozens of other things. If you're a woman, please refer to the section on ovarian cancer symptoms—even if you don't think you're at risk. You may be surprised by what you read.

CHAPTER 8

PEOPLE IN SPECIAL CIRCUMSTANCES

T here are hundreds of health conditions that affect the gastrointestinal tract. This chapter covers some of the more common disorders affecting the North American population, such as eating disorders; "woman stuff" ranging from normal symptoms of pregnancy to diseases such as endometriosis, pelvic inflammatory disease, and ovarian cancer; people with diabetes complications or thyroid disorders; seniors who are plagued by GI problems; and people with HIV. This chapter is not exhaustive but gives an idea of some of the other underlying causes of GI symptoms, referring you to other resources for more information.

WHEN YOU HAVE AN EATING DISORDER

There are several types of eating disorders, ranging from food refusal or starvation, known as anorexia nervosa, to bingeing and purging, known as binge eating disorder or bulimia nervosa. Two percent of the female population in North America suffers from one or the other, but experts estimate that the number is actually much higher than this; many women successfully hide these disorders for years. Eating disorders are diseases of control that mostly affect women. "Fat" is perceived as a public announcement that a person is "out of control." This perception becomes increasingly more distorted until the act of eating at all is perceived as a loss of control. Bulimics are said to be "failed anorexics"; their bingeing is a sign that they are not able to stay in control, while the purging is their way of regaining control of the situation. Anorexics are driven by fear of their own appetites. (Appetite for life—sex, love, desires, ambition—becomes entangled and twisted around appetite for food.)

A small percentage of people suffer from a physical disorder called achalasia, where muscles in the GI tract do not relax; this can cause vomiting or reflux. Such people may be labeled with an eating disorder, such as bulimia, when in fact they suffer from achalasia. If you believe you're being inaccurately diagnosed with bulimia nervosa, make sure your doctor takes an accurate history (see chapter 2) as well as the appropriate diagnostic tests to rule out a physical cause for chronic vomiting.

Anorexia Nervosa

This term means "loss of appetite due to mental disorder." It includes several starvation-related symptoms, ranging from skin disorders to cardiovascular problems. When it comes to GI symptoms, people with anorexia nervosa will experience symptoms of dysmotility (see chapter 4): feeling full after eating a few bites, abdominal fullness and bloating, gas, nausea, and possibly heartburn from poor functioning of the lower esophageal sphincter. Starvation causes the GI tract to slow down, causing a real, physical problem of dysmotility. The treatment in this case is the same used for anyone with dysmotility—a prokinetic agent such as cis-apride. Refer to chapters 4 and 5 for more details.

Some complications arise, however, when medical personnel don't believe that you're truly suffering from the dysmotility symptoms you describe. It is common for such symptoms to be misconstrued as psychological elements of a disease. In other words, it is assumed that you're saying "I'm full" or "I don't feel well" because you're afraid of food, not because real organic symptoms are at work, delaying gastric emptying. If you have dysmotility symptoms and your doctor does not believe you, insist on a referral to a gastroenterologist and tell the eating disorder specialist(s): "I'm not making this up just to avoid eating; in fact, I'm disclosing these symptoms to you so I can begin to recover and eat normal amounts of food comfortably. I believe I'm suffering from a motility problem, which I understand is a physical manifestation of my eating disorder." That ought to do the trick and get you the treatment you need for your dysmotility symptoms.

Constipation is another common problem experienced by recovering anorexics, caused by starvation. When the upper GI tract slows down, causing fullness and bloating, the lower region also slows down, delaying the passage of stools and solid waste. It's important to keep in mind that you may think you're constipated when you're experiencing a normal bowel pattern. For instance, when you're in the process of "refeeding" and just beginning to eat normally again, it may take about a week for your body to pass stool, as it's busy taking in nutrients from the food. Eating a proper diet high in fiber and liquids will help the problem enormously. If you're being treated for a motility problem with cisapride, your constipation will probably be relieved at the same time. It's crucial that you do *not* take a laxative, however. Allowing your colon to "reawaken" and begin functioning again is crucial.

Bulimia Nervosa

There are many kinds of purging behaviors seen in bulimia nervosa, which means "hunger like an ox due to mental disorder." The bingeing episodes are always followed by some sort of purging, which may include:

- self-induced vomiting
- abusing laxatives and/or diuretics
- misusing other drugs, including thyroid medication or insulin (Type 1 diabetic women may deliberately withhold their insulin to induce weight loss)
- overexercising

Bingeing and GI symptoms

Regardless of the purge method used, the binge episode by itself can cause symptoms such as abdominal bloating, distention, and fullness to the extent where breathlessness can occur, as the distended stomach presses up against the diaphragm. There are even documented cases of people requiring emergency surgery from tears (due to vomiting), causing bleeding or rupturing of the esophagus. The bingeing, of course, can also cause weight gain, putting you at risk for all the obesity-related conditions, such as cardiovascular problems, Type 2 diabetes, and gallbladder disease (see chapter 7).

Self-induced vomiting and GI symptoms

For the purposes of this chapter, self-induced vomiting refers to people who engage in this behavior on a chronic basis (one to three times per week or more). If you've self-induced vomiting only occasionally due to other circumstances, such as food poisoning, you are not in danger of developing any of these problems.

If you're a chronic purger/vomiter, the first place you'll notice GI symptoms is in your mouth. Vomit contains large amounts of stomach acid, which will erode the enamel off your teeth and cause dental problems and cavities. As your teeth become more exposed, you'll start to feel a sensitivity to hot and cold, which can usually be treated by brushing with a toothpaste such as Sensodyne and with a fluoride gel, which can help protect your teeth from further cavities. Immediately brushing with baking soda and flossing after a vomiting episode is recommended.

You may also notice that about a week after a purging episode, one of your salivary glands, the parotid gland, may swell (known as sialadenosis), which can give you "chipmunk" cheeks. Once you stop your vomiting, the glands should go back to their normal size. In the meantime, heat or sucking on tart fruits or candies can help.

Vomiting will also cause gastroesophageal reflux disease (GERD), chronic heartburn or "sour stomach," and all the symptoms discussed in chapter 4, as well as sores in the lining of the esophagus (see chapter 4), which may cause symptoms of vomiting bright red blood. In extreme cases, vomiting can also lead to tears in the mucosal lining of the esophagus, which is a serious condition that will also cause bleeding and vomiting blood. Forceful vomiting can also cause rupture of the esophagus, which is an extreme emergency. Severe chest pain that is brought on by breathing, yawning, or swallowing is a sign of an esophageal rupture, which is a very serious condition.

As a rule, if you're a chronic vomiter, be sure to have your blood checked for signs of anemia, which means that you could be suffering from internal bleeding. Other GI problems include dysphagia, or difficulty swallowing, as well as the loss of electrolytes and fluids, which can lead to cardiovascular failure in severe cases.

Treating GI problems related to chronic vomiting starts with treating the underlying problem: *stopping* the vomiting through an effective eating disorder treatment program. In the meantime, a gastroenterologist can perform tests to determine the extent of the damage to your GI tract and can prescribe acid-lowering drugs to help with the symptoms.

Laxative abuse

If you're abusing laxatives (and your doctor may have no idea), the first thing you need to understand is that you generally don't lose weight this way. That's because all the calories and nutrients are absorbed in the upper GI tract. By the time the food gets down to your colon, you're losing water and electrolytes, not calories. Stimulant laxatives stimulate the colon to contract, resulting in a bowel movement. Stimulant laxatives include senna (common in herbal laxatives), cascara (described as a "tonic" in some herbal books) and phenolphthalein, the common medicinal ingredient used in more than fifty over-the-counter laxatives, such as Ex-Lax, Phillips Gelcaps, and Carter's Little Liver Pills. Phenolphthalein is considered by the National Toxicology Program in the United States to be potentially carcinogenic; manufacturers have been ordered to stop selling laxatives with phenolphthalein as of this writing, unless the ingredient can be proved safe.

If a stimulant laxative is abused, the result can be cathartic colon syndrome, a condition where you're plagued with chronic constipation because the colon has lost its ability to contract without external stimulants. So, without a laxative, you'll feel abdominal bloating and swelling, which can be very uncomfortable.

The only way to treat laxative dependency is to go into a sort of detox program, where you adjust your diet (high fiber and fluid intake) and life-style (lots of exercise and patience) until your colonic function is restored. There are nonstimulant laxatives, such as lactulose; herbal preparations promoting regularity with herbs that are simply good for digestion, such as ginger, cumin, licorice root, and other spices, without senna or cascara, may be helpful.

For more information on eating disorders, consult the appendix of this book, as well as *The Eating Disorder Sourcebook* by Carolyn Costin.

"GI JANE"

"Just because you're a woman" is often a good enough reason for GI problems. It's not fair, but who said anatomy was fair? The challenge for women is to distinguish between gynecological disorders and true GI disorders. The general rule is to note how your symptoms correlate to your menstrual cycle and/or your sexual activity. For example, if you notice symptoms a few months after a new partner (with months of celibacy in between), you may have contracted a sexually transmitted disease—or you may be pregnant. If you always experience symptoms about two weeks before your period, then you may have PMS or endometriosis. If you experience abdominal pain after or during intercourse, your pain is likely to be connected to a gynecological problem.

PMS (Premenstrual Symptoms/Syndrome)

Few women have difficulty separating their PMS from a GI disorder. The hormonal symphony that controls your cycles can bring on a host of emotional and physical symptoms, usually beginning about two weeks prior to your period. Women report the following GI symptoms:

- weight gain and abdominal bloating
- constipation or diarrhea

▣ sugar and salt cravings and increased appetite

▣ nausea

How do you know when symptoms are PMS-related? They will usually go away once you get your period. If they don't, you should consult a gastroenterologist or family doctor to try to find the source of your symptoms. Treatments for PMS vary, but the most effective treatments revolve around adjusting intake of caffeine, sugar, and salt about fourteen days prior to your period. Several herbs and vitamins have been noted for helping to ease PMS symptoms as well. For more information, consult my book *The Gynecological Sourcebook*.

Pregnancy

In the physiology of pregnancy, smooth muscle relaxes to prevent the uterus from contracting during the nine months. Unfortunately, this can create a number of gastrointestinal symptoms, including gastroesophageal reflux disease (GERD), discussed in chapter 4, as well as constipation.

GERD is caused by two things. In early pregnancy, hormones can relax the lower esophageal sphincter; later in pregnancy, your expanding uterus presses up against the esophagus, interfering with the lower esophageal sphincter. The result in either case is heartburn. If you've suffered from GERD in the past, pregnancy often makes it worse. Morning sickness can also cause nausea and reflux, while many women will also be plagued with anal symptoms such as hemorrhoids (see chapter 6). Treatment for GI symptoms during pregnancy is "tea and sympathy." Various herbal teas may help with certain symptoms, but beyond that, taking any sort of medication during pregnancy is not recommended without strict permission from your doctor. For more information on pregnancy symptoms, consult my book *The Pregnancy Sourcebook*.

Endometriosis

The clinical definition of endometriosis is "abnormal growth of endometrial cells." The endometrium is the lining of the uterus, and endometriosis means that endometrial tissue grows outside the uterus within the general abdominal cavity. Sometimes mild endometriosis can cause severe symptoms, while severe endometriosis may cause only mild symptoms. In other words, the severity of symptoms does not correlate to the severity of the disease. Roughly 5.5 million women throughout North America have endometriosis.

Endometriosis includes so many seemingly unrelated symptoms, it's often missed or misdiagnosed. Here is a checklist of symptoms you should watch for. If you find you have at least two of these symptoms during your period or chronically, you may want to be checked for endometriosis.

- pelvic pain and/or painful intercourse (in one survey, 78 percent of women with endometriosis reported pain severe enough to wake them at night or else interfere with their falling asleep)
- infertility (this is often the only symptom women experience—even with Stage IV)
- abnormal cycles or periods
- nausea and/or vomiting
- exhaustion
- bladder problems
- frequent infections
- dizziness
- painful defecation
- lower backaches
- irritable bowels (loose, watery, and often bloody diarrhea; many women diagnosed with irritable bowel syndrome [IBS] really have endometriosis)

- other stomach problems
- low-grade fever

A questionnaire distributed by the Endometriosis Association revealed that 100 percent of respondents experienced pain one to two days prior to their periods. In addition, 71 percent reported pain mid-cycle; 40 percent reported pain at other times; 20 percent reported pain throughout their cycle, while 7 percent reported intermittent pain with no particular pattern. The pain in this questionnaire was mostly abdominal pain. It's common for women with endometriosis to be diagnosed and treated for conditions they really don't have. This occurs because of the confusing group of symptoms that characterize endometriosis. In some cases, symptoms may mimic irritable bowel syndrome (discussed in chapter 6) or a host of other ailments.

Experts recommend that if you suspect you have endometriosis, you should request that a pelvic exam be performed during your period, when endometriosis is in full "flare." This may help your doctor to find certain clues that will send you in the right diagnostic direction. For example, transvaginal ultrasound versus abdominal ultrasound is very useful in finding many of the physical clues that endometriosis leaves behind, such as cysts or masses. You may want to request a transvaginal ultrasound even when your doctor doesn't order it.

There is a sister condition to endometriosis known as adenomyosis, which has similar symptoms. An enlarged, soft, or tender uterus is a classic sign of adenomyosis.

Pelvic Inflammatory Disease (PID)

PID is caused by two sexually transmitted diseases: chlamydia and gonorrhea. Many times, women with PID are infected with both. What happens is that these infections travel up the pelvic tract, causing scarring and inflammation. The symptoms are usually lower abdominal pain, frequently on one side (which means a fallopian tube may be involved), which increases when you move around (walking, climbing, etc.). Other PID symptoms may manifest as painful bowel movements, a continuous feeling that you have to move your bowels, abdominal bloating, nausea and dizziness, and general malaise.

This is all quite vague. If you're suffering from any of these symptoms, see your doctor and make sure you note whether you've had unprotected sex with anyone new in the past few months. Antibiotics will cure PID, but there may be long-term consequences, such as infertility due to blocked tubes (which can be treated). For more information on PID and infertility, consult my books *The Gynecological Sourcebook* and *The Fertility Sourcebook*.

Ovarian Cancer Symptoms

A book on GI disorders may be a more appropriate place to discuss ovarian cancer than a book on women's health. That's because the symptoms of ovarian cancer are GI—not gynecological. This is a deadly cancer for women because 70 percent of cases are found at an advanced stage. This is because the symptoms are so vague and gastrointestinal in nature that few women suspect it's cancer at all—let alone a gynecological cancer. However, if discovered early, ovarian cancer carries an 85 to 95 percent five-year survival rate.

Going for regular pelvic exams and watching for the following GI symptoms will help you catch this cancer before it's too late.

Alarm symptoms in women over fifty
- Symptoms of GERD (heartburn, bloating, feeling full early in a meal, gas, and other symptoms discussed in chapter 4)
- discomfort in the lower abdomen

- painless swelling or bloating in the lower abdomen
- loss of appetite
- gas and indigestion
- nausea
- weight loss
- constipation
- pain during intercourse

These symptoms are particularly alarming when you have . . .

- a family history of breast, ovarian, or colorectal cancer
- never been pregnant
- taken fertility drugs in the past
- been exposed to environmental toxins
- had irregular periods
- a high-fat, low-fiber diet

If you have two or more of these symptoms, go to your doctor and say: "I want you to feel for an enlarged ovary or mass." If this doesn't reveal anything, discuss the merits of other investigational procedures such as transvaginal pelvic ultrasound to rule out ovarian cancer. When it comes to this kind of deadly cancer, better safe than sorry. Again, consult my book *The Gynecological Sourcebook* for more information.

IF YOU HAVE DIABETES

People with diabetes, especially Type 1 or insulin-dependent diabetes, are susceptible to what's called diabetic neuropathy, or nerve disease. High blood sugar levels can affect the nerves that control the entire gastrointestinal tract. As a result, you could suffer from dysmotility, discussed in chapter 4, which will affect gastric emptying. Not only will you experience general abdominal discomfort and bloating, but when your stomach doesn't empty, it's hard to regulate your insulin, which can lead to other problems.

Roughly 60 percent of the nerve damage associated with Type 1 diabetes can be prevented by achieving tight control over blood sugar levels. This involves frequent blood sugar monitoring with a home glucose test kit to check postmeal blood sugar levels, and adjusting food intake and exercise regimen to accommodate the readings. Motility problems may be controlled with diet and life-style adjustment and possibly a prokinetic agent such as cisapride. For more information, contact the American or Canadian Diabetes Association.

IF YOU HAVE THYROID DISEASE

The thyroid gland is a butterfly-shaped gland situated in front of the windpipe. It secretes thyroid hormone, which regulates metabolism. When the thyroid gland is overactive, known as hyperthyroidism (there are many causes), it makes too much thyroid hormone. Therefore, the entire body speeds up—particularly the gastrointestinal tract. In this case, your appetite would increase yet you'd be losing weight. Bowel movements may become more frequent and looser, or you may notice diarrhea. Other symptoms of hyperthyroidism include an enlarged thyroid gland, a fast pulse or heart palpitations, irritability, an intolerance to heat (i.e., you feel hot all the time), as well as bulging of the eyes or vision problems.

When the thyroid gland is underactive, known as hypothyroidism, the GI tract is slowed down. You'll suffer from constipation, hardening of stools, bloating, poor appetite, as well as heartburn and weight gain. Other symptoms of hypothyroidism include extreme fatigue, an enlarged thyroid gland, skin changes, hair loss, and poor memory and concentration.

If thyroid disease runs in your family, you're especially vulnerable to it. A good rule is to request a thyroid function test when you notice the recent onset of these symptoms. For more information, consult my book *The Thyroid Sourcebook*.

IF YOU'RE OVER SIXTY-FIVE

Seniors and GI disorders go hand in hand. As we age, our GI tract can slow down unless we are eating sufficient amounts of fiber and getting enough exercise. The other problem is that many seniors are taking several medications simultaneously, many of which are constipating.

Cardiovascular medications can contribute to heartburn/reflux symptoms, as well as dysmotility, weakening the lower esophageal sphincter pressure. Before taking any specific GI drug, it's important to review with your doctor all the medications you're taking. You may be able to adjust or stop certain medications and thereby solve your GI problems. However, because you're in an age group that's at higher risk for cancer, you should also have a thorough workup (see chapter 2) to investigate your GI symptoms.

Ultimately, getting some exercise and practicing a low-fat, high-fiber, and high-fluid diet will help to prevent or alleviate GI symptoms, such as constipation or heartburn. If you're juggling many different medications and are experiencing GI problems, you may wish to consult with a gerontologist, a physician who specializes in treating the myriad of health problems facing the senior population.

WHEN YOU'RE HIV-POSITIVE

This section discusses common opportunistic infections that are considered to be AIDS-defining illnesses in people who are HIV-positive. However, these problems are uncommon in people who are newly infected with HIV who are on preventive combination drug therapies. For more information on the conditions discussed below, contact the Gay Men's Health Crisis (women are also welcome!) at (212) 807-7035 or any of the AIDS organizations listed in your area. The GMHC has exceptionally good literature available, mailed out free of charge in plain envelopes.

Oral Thrush

Roughly 80 percent of all HIV-positive persons who have progressed to a more serious stage of illness will experience oral thrush, which is oral candidiasis—yeast. Here, the tongue becomes coated in a milky white goop that looks terrible but isn't life-threatening. You may also experience burning or stinging. Thrush sometimes occurs in HIV-negative people who are on antibiotics or cortisone. Diabetics may also develop thrush. Oral thrush, however, never develops unless there is some kind of medical problem.

Thrush is treated with topical nystatin or clotrimazole (Mycelex) lozenges. Ketoconazole (Nizoral), available in pill form, is also used, and you can now get oral fluconazole (Diflucan) and itraconazole as well. Nutritionists or naturopaths can also recommend a diet that can help ward off thrush.

Myobacterium Aviumintracellular Complex (MAC)

MAC is really an atypical form of tuberculosis, but it may or may not cause chest or respiratory symptoms. It doesn't develop until the body's T-cells are fewer than fifty. If you do develop a cough, however, the cough is less severe than in TB, but you will suffer from severe gastrointestinal symptoms. Symptoms of MAC include weight loss, chronic high fever, severe anemia, chills and night sweats, abdominal pain, chronic diarrhea, swollen lymph nodes, reduction in white blood cells (neutropenia), and an enlarged liver and spleen.

General Weight Loss

Weight loss can occur when oral infections make eating difficult. If the body does not get enough calories from the diet, it takes them out of the proteins in the muscles. (See Tables 8.1 and 8.2.) Some other causes of weight loss include:

- **Depression** (Appetite loss is a symptom of biological depression and can be treated with appetite stimulants such as Megace and Marinol [oral marijuana], or liquid supplements.)
- **Fever** (First, treat the underlying cause of the fever; next, ask your doctor for an appropriate fever reducer. Don't self-treat, as many fever reducers conflict with other medications.)
- **Diarrhea** (Can be relieved with Imodium, Kaopectate, or stronger drugs. Experts also suggest Gatorade to replace lost electrolytes; avoid eating seeds, bran, nuts, whole-wheat bread, the skins of fruits and vegetables, dairy products, and caffeine. A diet of bananas, rice, applesauce/juice, and tea—dubbed the BRAT diet—is the general rule.)

Wasting

Wasting is an involuntary weight loss of 10 percent or more of the body weight. Infectious diarrhea or parasitic infections are usually responsible for wasting. The treatment is to find the cause and/or treat the symptoms. For example, if wasting is caused by loss of appetite or diarrhea, dietary supplementation is the treatment. If nausea and vomiting are the cause, small, frequent, bland meals may be the best treatment, along with nausea-control medications. In more severe cases, tube feeding or intravenous feeding may be necessary.

Oral Hairy Leukoplakia (OHL)

This is an oral infection caused by the Epstein Barr virus and is characterized by white patches on the tongue and/or in adjacent areas in the mouth, and microscopic "hair" forming on the tongue's surface. These white patches can be as thick as an inch and can coat most of the tongue. A sore mouth and sometimes

TABLE 8.1 **Foods to Avoid if You're HIV-Positive**

- Raw or undercooked meat (especially pork)

- Raw seafood (sushi, oysters, etc.)

- Raw eggs (in homemade mayonnaise, for example), as well as eggs—poached, boiled, scrambled, or fried—that are not thoroughly cooked

- Luncheon meats made from a variety of unspecified meats and fillers

- Unwashed or broken-skinned fruits and vegetables

- Unpasteurized milk and milk products

- Leftovers after the second day (due to an increase in bacterial growth)

- Foods with an excessive fat content (although often suggested as a remedy for AIDS wasting syndrome, this approach actually defeats the purpose because the high-fat content aggravates diarrhea)

- Foods that have been left unrefrigerated for long periods of time or have been prepared under unsanitary or questionable conditions (such as items sold by street vendors)

Source: Adapted from Patricia Kloser and Jane MacLean Craig, The Woman's HIV Sourcebook (Dallas: M. S. Taylor, 1994), pp. 51–52.

TABLE 8.2 **Combating Eating Problems**
Following are some suggestions for effectively coping with various eating problems that plague the HIV-infected or people undergoing cancer therapy.

- Pain/difficulty swallowing:

  Try such soft foods as mashed potatoes; scrambled eggs with cheese; yogurt; cottage cheese; custards; flaked fish; ground meat; tuna, egg, or chicken salad; in addition to a liquid supplement specially formulated for people with HIV. If problems are severe, food may be put through a blender or baby food may be eaten. Avoid salty, spicy, and "rough" foods, such as raw vegetables and all citrus fruits. To prevent the irritation of ultrasensitive tissue in the mouth, the temperature of foods should not be too hot.

- Diarrhea:

  Bananas, applesauce, rice, and plenty of liquids should be consumed to replace lost fluids. Gatorade or Gastrolyte, which is similar to Pedialyte (sold in the infant department of pharmacies), will help replace electrolytes depleted by diarrhea.

- Nausea:

  Eat crackers, dry toast, pretzels, or bland cookies (arrowroot biscuits or vanilla wafers, for example). Also try cold foods like chicken or tuna salad, and cottage cheese with fruit. Avoid spicy, greasy foods as well as those with a strong odor. If vomiting occurs, maintain a liquids-only diet, consisting of clear broth, apple juice, tea, and ginger ale. Jell-O and popsicles are also usually well tolerated. Ask your doctor to prescribe an antinausea medication.

- Loss of appetite:

  Some prescription appetite stimulants (such as Megace or Marinol) are effective under such circumstances, so speak to your doctor about prescribing one for you. In addition, make your meals small, frequent, and dense in calories and protein. Try doing some form of relaxation exercise twenty to thirty minutes before eating.

Source: Adapted from Patricia Kloser and Jane MacLean Craig, The Woman's HIV Sourcebook (Dallas: M. S. Taylor, 1994), pp. 53–54.

changes in the voice can also develop. This is often misdiagnosed as thrush, but will not respond to thrush treatment. The treatment for OHL is high doses of acyclovir, taken in pill or capsule form.

Cytomegalovirus Infection (CMV)

This is a virus that half the population carries but never worries about. However, with HIV infection, CMV can cause a host of problems, including abnormal vision (CMV retinitis); pneumonia (CMV pneumonitis); hepatitis (CMV hepatitis); colitis (CMV colitis); fever and fatigue; and brain inflammation (CMV cerebritis). CMV doesn't usually develop until the late stages of AIDS. Treatment for all the above conditions involves the intravenous drug ganciclovir or foscarnet, used alone or in conjunction with gancyclovir.

Cryptosporidiosis

This is a contagious parasite that causes a severe form of watery diarrhea with ten to twenty bowel movements a day. It can be diagnosed through a stool exam. Treatment depends on its severity and whether fever and abdominal pains accompany it.

A Word to Caregivers

It's a good idea to wear disposable surgical gloves when handling bodily fluids of someone with HIV. The virus can be transmitted through cuts and abrasions on the hands or arms, and so urine, vomit, diarrhea, or blood can infect you. You may also want to wear disposable medical gowns when handling bodily fluids.

If the person you are caring for has an active cough, she or he should be wearing a mask to prevent the spread of TB (even if you're not sure whether it is TB). If you have a cold or cough, you should wear a mask to protect your loved one.

All used tissues, soiled bandages, dressings, gloves, pads, and tampons should be disposed of immediately in sealed plastic bags. They should then be tossed into a trash can with a secure lid.

All washable surfaces should be cleaned with a solution of one-half cup bleach to one gallon of water, and then rinsed well with plain water.

Each time you touch your loved one or handle his or her bodily fluids, wash your hands in warm soapy water and then rinse (even if you're wearing gloves). Make sure you use a moisturizing lotion on your hands to help prevent them from chapping or cracking.

This chapter touches only briefly upon the groups of people who may experience GI symptoms as side effects or complications of other disorders. It's worth noting that stress (discussed briefly in chapter 6) can interfere with the entire GI tract. While under stress, your body produces chemicals known as catecholamines, which can lead to dysmotility (see chapter 4), IBS, and episodes of vomiting. Any chronic disease can cause stress, which may exacerbate the GI complications caused by the organic nature of the disease itself.

It's also important to note that if you're having chemotherapy to treat any kind of cancer, you will no doubt experience GI problems. Chemotherapy usually causes nausea and vomiting that subsides a few days after the treatment cycle. Antinausea drugs can alleviate some of these symptoms. External or internal radiation to the lower back or lower abdominal region will almost certainly cause tenderness and diarrhea, which can be helped with antidiarrheal drugs. Meanwhile, external radiation to the neck or throat area will make swallowing difficult. Topical anesthetics can be used in this case to ease swallowing.

The next chapter will unveil the secrets to living well, and will also tell you what you can do to help prevent all kinds of cancers—colorectal cancer in particular.

CHAPTER 9

EATING WELL, FEELING WELL

The secret to living well and feeling well is eating well. This translates into a diet high in fiber and low in fat. Researchers have also found that adopting this type of diet can dramatically reduce the incidence of colorectal cancer, heart disease, stroke, and obesity-related conditions, ranging from gallbladder disease to Type 2 diabetes.

Exercise is also a crucial component to feeling well. Numerous studies show that people who do some form of nonstop aerobic activity for twenty minutes three times per week have much lower rates of disease. Finally, eating well combined with appropriate levels of exercise won't get you very far if you're a smoker. Smoking is hard on the lungs, heart . . . and GI tract.

This chapter will discuss current theories in disease prevention and wellness. I'll explain how to cut dietary fat, increase fiber, and how to interpret some of the newfangled food terms, such as *phytochemicals* and *functional foods*, that are splashing across the health pages. The section entitled "How to Prevent Colon Cancer Without Really Trying" explains how you can maintain your lower intestinal fortitude by simply eating a variety of vegetables and grains—crucial reading for anyone over forty-five who is at risk for colon cancer, outlined in chapter 6.

....

WHAT HISTORY TEACHES US

The word *diet* comes from the Greek word *diatta,* which means "way of life." In more modern times the word *diet* has come to be associated with a narrower definition, such as weight loss or a restricted eating regimen. The term *diatta* obviously has much broader implications, as many religions tell us when they incorporate dietary rules into their life-styles and faiths.

Many of us are eating the wrong things and eating too much. As society became more advanced and the Industrial Revolution brought about widespread changes in food technology, we began to see more modern diseases, such as stomach ailments and cancers. In fact, these diseases are linked by many nutritionists to the invention of refined flour and changes in water supply.

We also know that cancer rates are higher in the United States than in Asia, but that genetics seems to have little to do with it. Are we eating something we shouldn't, or are Asians eating some foods that we should eat? Or, do they stop eating certain foods when they emigrate to the West, and this accounts for the difference? For example, Japanese diets average roughly 15 percent calories from fat; American diets average about 40 percent fat. The traditional Japanese diet of rice, vegetables, and fish is far different from the meat, fat, and sugar of North American diets.

Nevertheless, everyone agrees that the Western diet is unhealthy; it contains more calories, fat, and meat than other diets, leading to heart disease, stroke, and the development of colorectal and other cancers. Epidemiologists know that cultures that stick to a traditional diet of whole grains, cooked vegetables, and fresh seasonal fruit have less cancer.

Overnutrition

Hippocrates referred to cancer in general as a disease of overnutrition. When you look at today's statistics, he may have been onto something. The "refiner" things in life, such as sugar, white flour, and other processed foods—coupled with excess protein and fat—contribute to a number of diseases. For proof, just take a look at any pharmacy shelf and survey the antacids and constipation remedies available.

For thousands of years, cooked whole grains were considered a dietary staple. In the Orient this meant rice and millet; in Europe it meant wheat, oats, and rye; in Russia, buckwheat; in Africa, sorghum; in the Middle East, barley; and in the Americas, corn (prior to the white man's invasion).

Of course, a diet based on grains is nonexistent in the West today. We consume, by any standards, an obscene amount of meat. The proof is in statistics put out by the U.S. Department of Agriculture (USDA). Between 1910 and 1976, wheat consumption dropped by 48 percent; corn by 85 percent; rye by 78 percent; barley by 66 percent; buckwheat by 98 percent; beans and legumes by 46 percent; fresh vegetables by 23 percent; and fresh fruit by 33 percent. Meanwhile, the consumption of beef rose by 72 percent; poultry by 194 percent; cheese by 322 percent; canned vegetables by 320 percent; frozen vegetables by 1,650 percent; processed fruit by 556 percent; and soft drinks by 2,638 percent. And since 1940, chemical additives and preservatives in our food have risen by 995 percent.

In its report on the impact of modern farming and food processing, The American Association of Advancement of Science stated that a diet centered on whole-grain cereals and vegetables rather than meat, poultry, and so on, would benefit our entire way of life, making more land, water, fuel, and mineral use available. This, in turn, would have positive effects on inflation, employment, and international trade.

THE MEANING OF LOW-FAT

There are three different kinds of fats (technically called fatty acids): saturated, monounsaturated, and polyunsaturated. How saturated a fat is has to do with the number of hydrogen atoms in the fat molecule. Hydrogen is what makes fat solid, as in butter or lard. Unsaturated fats are more liquid, as in oils.

When a company wants to market a spread, such as margarine, by using 100 percent pure unsaturated fats, it needs to add hydrogen to the unsaturated fat to make it more solid; this process is called hydrogenation, which creates the fat equivalent of a transvestite. The resulting product is known as a transfatty acid; although sold as an unsaturated fat, it is treated like a saturated fat by the body because of its hydrogenation.

Lowering fat content in the diet means primarily cutting out all saturated fat and replacing it, in moderation, with unsaturated fat—which can actually be good for you. Research shows that the healthiest diets are those in which only 20 percent of calories come from fat.

Cholesterol and Fat

The reason why you want to lower your intake of saturated fat is that you want to decrease your level of low-density lipids, or "bad cholesterol." Low-density lipoproteins (LDL) are the artery-clogging substances that can cause cardiovascular problems—heart disease or stroke. High-density lipids (HDL), or the "good cholesterol," will not clog arteries. This is the type of cholesterol that your body is happy to have around, and it is necessary in order for your liver to make bile (see chapter 7) and steroid hormones. In fact, more HDL is increasingly seen as more desirable. Studies show that the more HDL in your blood, the lower your risk of developing cardiovascular problems. HDL apparently carries cholesterol out of the blood and back to the liver for breakdown and excretion.

Saturated fats (tropical oils or animal fat) raise LDL levels (and sometimes lower HDL levels); in fact, they stimulate the body to make cholesterol. Meanwhile, mono- and polyunsaturated fats raise HDL levels, and may even decrease LDL levels. Olive oil is an example of a "good fat"—a polyunsaturated one.

Fish oils, found in coldwater fish such as salmon, mackerel, sable, whitefish, herring, and sardines, are very high sources of omega-3 oils, highly polyunsaturated fats that are said to offer protection from heart disease.

Cancer and Fat

Many studies have been trying to show a connection between cancer and dietary fat. Until quite recently, the only cancer that researchers agreed was reduced by lower-fat diets was colon cancer, which I'll go into further on. Most recently, environmental scientists such as Dr. Sandra Steingraber, author of *Living Downstream: An Ecologist Looks at Cancer and the Environment,* points out that body fat is a host for environmental toxins. The more fat in your body, the more inviting you make it for carcinogenic toxins to move in and wreak havoc on healthy cells. These toxins range from pesticides to a long list of other organochlorines. This is why lower-fat diets are associated with lower cancer rates of all kinds. Steingraber uses undisputed examples of toxins living in fat by explaining why beluga whales get bladder cancer and breast cancer. (You certainly can't accuse whales of smoking, drinking, or not exercising!)

How to detox your food

The best place to start the environmental cleanup is in your kitchen. Your weekly groceries probably contain residues from pesticides and other organochlorines on store-bought fruits and vegetables; hormones in meat products; as well as a number of extras you may not have bargained for, which were fed to your meat when it was still alive. These include feed additives, antibiotics, and tranquilizers. Meanwhile, anything packaged will most likely contain dyes and flavors from a variety of chemical concoctions.

Airborne contaminants, waste, and spills affect the water and soil, which in turn affect virtually everything we ingest. In addition, when one species becomes unable to reproduce, the food chain is interrupted, and the problem eventually trickles down to our kitchen tables. Cleaning up the food chain is all part of creating a healthy, contaminant-free diet for ourselves. You can find out what your produce has eaten, and whether it was injected with anything, by calling the USDA information line at (202) 720-2791. (Canadians can call Agriculture and Agrafood Canada at [613] 952-8000.) The USDA can also tell you where your fish has swum and what your produce was sprayed with.

Since the origin of the word *consumer* comes from the word *consume*—to eat—becoming vigilant about our groceries is the only way to help change the produce and food industry. Customers are incredibly important to any company. In the 1980s, it was the "vigilante consumer" who helped to make manufacturers more green-friendly and value-conscious. In many instances, the sheer volume of customer complaints and letters has completely changed not only individual companies' habits and policies, but an entire industry. If enough customers ban products, protest manufacturing or agricultural practices, and so on, the companies will change. Bring new meaning to the adage "The customer is always right"!

Worried about the toxicity of the soil your vegetables were grown in? Demand labeling that identifies the contents of that soil. Write letters to manufacturers; call 800 numbers; start a newsgroup on the Internet; lobby; protest; ban products to help change standards. "What was this spinach sprayed with?" You have a right to a label that reads: "This produce sprayed with endosulfan."

Milking the System

If you are lactose intolerant, you may discover that you're not missing much. As adults, we actually don't need milk, even though we consume obscene quantities of it in North America. Within the United States, each person consumes roughly 350 pounds of milk per year, which is equal to roughly 72 gallons. That translates into one cow for every second person. However, because of the heating procedures, homogenization, sterilization, addition of other ingredients such as vitamin D, hormones, antibodies, and other chemicals in milk, many people question whether it's still nature's perfect food. When you consider that 75 percent of all dairy cows are artificially inseminated, milk somehow loses its wholesome appeal.

The interesting thing about modern milk is that before we were able to store and preserve milk, most of the dairy products consumed were limited to fermented dairy foods, such as yogurt and kefir, which contain enzymes and bacteria that help us break down lactose.

Animal milk (goat, sheep, or donkey) was once reserved for mothers who could not breast-feed, but the huge quantities of cow's milk humans ingest today were never intended by nature.

By simply cutting down on your dietary dairy fat, you can do a lot to reduce your intake of saturated fat. Here's what you need to know to make some changes:

- Whole milk gets 48 percent of its calories from fat
- 2% milk gets 37 percent of its calories from fat
- 1% milk gets 26 percent of its calories from fat
- Skim milk is completely fat-free
- Cheese gets 50 percent of its calories from fat, unless it's made from skim milk
- Butter gets 95 percent of its calories from fat
- Yogurt gets 15 percent of its calories from fat

More Ways to Skim the Fat

The best way to cut your dietary fat is simply to read labels carefully. A product that boasts fewer calories can mean anything from low sodium to low sugar, but not necessarily fewer fat grams. Products that boast of being "lower" in fat need to be compared to something. For example, anything may be lower in fat than lard or butter. If you read a label that boasts "No cholesterol," this probably means the product contains no animal fats, but it could contain saturated fats, such as vegetable oil, which will raise your cholesterol levels anyway. Some of the most fattening products are sold as health foods: granola bars (200 calories with roughly 50 percent derived from fat), carob, and yogurt candies. Even low-fat frozen yogurt can be high in fat—especially if you top it with fattening goodies.

Broiled, baked, steamed, poached, roasted, or microwaved foods are healthier than fried or deep-fried foods. Here are some more fat-fighting tips:

- Whenever you refrigerate animal fat (as in soups, stews, or curry dishes), skim the fat from the top before reheating and serving. A gravy skimmer will also help skim fats; the spout pours from the bottom, which helps the oils and fats to coagulate on top.

- To cut some fat out of canned goods (soups, tuna, etc.), pour the contents through a coffee filter first. You can also refrigerate the can first, which will make the fat rise to the top, so you can skim it off prior to serving.

- Substitutes for butter include yogurt (great on potatoes), low-fat cottage cheese, and jams and jellies. You can also blend half butter with half olive or canola oil to create your own lower-calorie spread. Or, at dinner, dip your bread into olive oil with some garlic, Italian style. For sandwiches, any condiment without butter, margarine, or mayonnaise is fine—mustards, yogurt, etc.

- Powdered nonfat milk is in vogue again—high in calcium, low in fat. Substitute it in any recipe calling for milk or cream.

- Experiment with fruit recipes for dessert. Things like sorbet with low-fat yogurt topping can still be elegant.

- Season low-fat foods well. That way, you won't miss the flavor of fat.

- Good carbohydrates are products with polysaccharide glucose (cereal grains, veggies, beans); bad carbohydrates are monosaccharide or disaccharide sugars (fruit, honey, dairy foods, refined sugar, other sweeteners). Use this information to make better choices.

- Good protein comes from vegetable sources (whole grains and bean products); bad proteins come from animal sources. Again, use this information to make better choices.

- Substitute low-fat turkey meat for red meat. It's a good start.

FIBERSPACE

Fiber is the part of a plant our bodies can't digest. This may sound like a bad thing, but in fact it's a good thing. Increasing fiber intake means two things: eating foods high in soluble fiber (which dissolves in water) as well as eating foods high in insoluble fiber (which absorbs water). Soluble fiber lowers LDL levels, or "bad cholesterol," by trapping fatty acids, according to one theory. Insoluble fiber doesn't affect cholesterol level, but it regulates bowel movements. Insoluble fiber decreases the "transit time" by increasing colon motility and limiting the time dietary toxins "hang around" the intestinal wall. This is why it can dramatically decrease the risk of colon cancer. As insoluble fiber moves through the digestive tract, it absorbs water like a sponge and helps stools form faster, which makes them softer and easier to pass.

Give peas a chance—as well as other legumes (dried beans). They are excellent sources of soluble fiber, as are soy, oats, carrots, oranges, bananas, and other fruits.

Good sources of insoluble fiber are wheat bran and whole grains, skins from various fruits and vegetables, seeds, leafy greens, and cruciferous vegetables (cauliflower, broccoli, brussels sprouts).

Phytochemicals and Functional Foods

In general, all green vegetables—such as broccoli, green beans, spinach, and lettuces—are good for cellular repair. All red, orange, yellow, and purple vegetables contain antioxidants—thought to be cancer-fighting substances.

Nutritional scientists have been slowly uncovering hidden treasures in vegetables that are believed to help fight diseases. These are called phytochemicals, or plant chemicals (*phyto* is Greek for "plant").

Lycopene, for example, which is found in tomatoes, red grapefruit, and red peppers, is thought to reduce the risk of certain cancers (the latest buzz is prostate cancer). Therefore, tomatoes can be labeled "functional foods" because they contain lycopene.

Functional foods are those that have significant levels of biologically active disease-preventing or health-promoting properties. In fact, in the near future, you may even see spaghetti sauce with a label that reads: "May reduce risk of prostate cancer." Quaker Oats now carries labeling that says it "May reduce the risk of heart disease" because oats and oat bran are high sources of soluble fiber.

In Europe, it's now popular to consume foods that improve the quality of microflora in the intestines (dubbed the "good gut bacteria"). In some countries, fermented milk products enhanced with lactobacilli and bifidobacteria are all the rage. In Japan, for example, a group of sugars have been found to improve intestinal microflora and decrease the risk of tooth decay when used as a sugar substitute. Therefore they are a popular functional food item.

Dozens of phytochemicals have been identified, ranging from isoflavones (found in soybeans) to saponins (found in spinach, potatoes, tomatoes, and oats).

These complicated labels may make it seem that it is difficult to obtain healthy nutrients. It's not. Eating a variety of fruits, grains, and vegetables will ensure that you are getting all the vitamins, nutrients, and phytochemicals your body needs.

HOW TO PREVENT COLON CANCER WITHOUT REALLY TRYING

By lowering fat and increasing fiber, you'll greatly reduce your risk of colon cancer. No cancer expert will dispute this, even though they can dispute the fat-fiber connection when it comes to other malignancies, such as breast cancer. In fact, it's estimated that by simply following a low-fat/high-fiber diet, you can avoid 90 percent of all stomach and colon cancers and 20 percent of gallbladder, pancreas, mouth, pharynx, and esophageal cancers. Diet may even play a role in preventing lung cancer; recent studies show that people with low intakes of carotene (orange, red, and purple plant foods) have higher rates of lung cancer.

Weight of Evidence

Of all the studies done on cancer and dietary fat, the strongest connections can be made between high-fat diets and colon cancer. In other words, people who consume high quantities of fat have higher rates of colon cancer. People who consume low quantities of fat have lower rates of colon cancer.

As for fiber, studies show that people who consume high quantities of fiber have lower rates of colon cancer, while people who consume low quantities of fiber have higher rates of colon cancer.

Studies also show that the amount of calories in the diet—regardless of whether they're from fat or fiber—can also increase the risk of colon cancer. One study found that in people under sixty-seven years of age, an extra 500 calories a day can increase colon cancer risk in men by 15 percent and in women by 11 percent.

The Vitamins

It's believed that fruits and vegetables high in antioxidants, phytoestrogens (plant estrogens, found in soy), and lignins may also protect against a variety of cancers—particularly estrogen-related cancers, such as breast. For example, vitamin A and beta-carotene are associated with preventing or even reversing lung, larynx, colon, prostate, bladder, stomach, esophageal, and possibly breast cancer. Vitamins C and E and selenium are associated, in particular, with low rates of stomach and esophageal cancers. It's believed that vitamins C and E block the formation of carcinogenic compounds in the stomach.

Why does your stomach have carcinogenic compounds in the first place? Many of these compounds come from nitrates and nitrite salts, which are found in vegetables, drinking water, fruit juices, cured meat, baked goods, and cereals. In many cases, these salts form nitrosamines and nitrosamides, substances that are thought to potentially cause stomach and esophageal cancers.

Studies also show that cruciferous vegetables, such as cabbage, brussels sprouts, cauliflower, and broccoli contain phytochemicals that protect against colon cancer.

PREVENTING COMMON GI PROBLEMS

Coming full circle, cutting fat and increasing fiber can alleviate several of the GI problems discussed in this book, not including ulcers (see chapter 3), ulcerative colitis, and Crohn's disease (see chapter 6).

Cutting fat will help you lose weight, which is a great help in reducing the risk of gallbladder disease (see chapter 7) and in easing symptoms of NUD or GERD (discussed in chapter 4). GERD sufferers should also cut out caffeine, peppermint, alcohol, citrus or acidic fruits, and pepper. Eating smaller meals, avoiding food at night, and going for a walk after a meal instead of lying down or sitting on the couch, will also help reduce symptoms.

People plagued by irritable bowel syndrome (IBS) usually report an improvement in their symptoms after adopting a high-fiber diet.

Will You Quit It?

On the flip side, practically all GI problems are worsened or even triggered by smoking. For one thing, smoking seems to change how food is generally processed by the body, inhibiting the absorption of various nutrients. Smoking can lead to GERD because it weakens the lower esophageal sphincter (discussed in chapters 2 and 4), and it can lead to dysmotility (see chapter 4) because it interferes with gastric emptying. As for ulcers (discussed in chapter 3), studies show that they take longer to heal in smokers than in nonsmokers.

The liver (see chapter 7) is also affected by smoking. Research suggests that smoking may interfere with the way the liver processes drugs and alcohol. There is also evidence that smoking increases the accumulation of bile salts in the stomach, which can make stomach acid harder to digest—particularly if you are experiencing symptoms of heartburn/reflux. Smoking may also aggravate cirrhosis of the liver.

Smoking also reduces the bicarbonate produced by the pancreas (see chapter 7), which prevents acid in the duodenum from being neutralized. Meanwhile, smokers tend to produce excess stomach acid.

The good news is that if you quit smoking, a lot of the digestive upset can be repaired. Even liver damage disappears once you stop smoking. (See Table 9.1.)

Wash Your Hands

This may seem like an unnecessary piece of advice, but it's amazing how many infectious GI diseases can be avoided by the simple act of washing your hands prior to eating and after going to the bathroom—especially in a public place. Some elementary schools are working a scheduled hand-washing program into their curriculum. An interesting study found that hand washing

TABLE 9.1   **How to Minimize Upper GI Symptoms**

1. Eat smaller, well-balanced, regular meals.

2. Avoid excessive amounts of:
   - fatty/fried foods
   - spicy foods
   - chocolate
   - caffeine
   - citrus juices
   - acidic fruits and vegetables
   - peppermint or spearmint
   - carbonated beverages
   - any other food that appears to produce discomfort for you

3. Stop smoking.

4. Lose weight and avoid tight-fitting clothes.

5. Whenever possible avoid:
   - ASA (aspirin)
   - Vitamin C
   - Anticholinergics
   - NSAIDs

6. Do the following when heartburn/regurgitation are predominant symptoms:
   - Wait at least 2 hours after meals before lying down
   - Avoid bedtime snacks
   - Elevate the head of the bed (15 cm or 6 inches)

Source: Patient information, Janssen Pharmaceutica, Inc., 1996.

in school at least four scheduled times a day led to fewer absences due to communicable illnesses—particularly gastrointestinal illnesses such as diarrhea-related diseases. Hand washing, in fact, reduced gastrointestinal diseases in one school by 60 percent.

Hospitals are also practicing much more rigid hand-washing practices, noticing, too, the reduction in gastrointestinal problems, such as abdominal pain, diarrhea, and vomiting.

The next chapter discusses the difficult journey ahead for those of you facing cancer of the gastrointestinal tract. While there are several different types of GI cancers, all cancer patients go through a universal experience: educating themselves.

CHAPTER 10

CANCER IN THE GI TRACT

This chapter takes you through the journey of being diagnosed with cancer in the GI tract. It provides a nontechnical explanation of what cancer actually is and the various types of GI cancer that can develop; it also explains the various stages of cancer and the system doctors use to tell what stage your cancer is in. It is not intended to provide details on GI cancer specifically; rather, it focuses on questions and answers that *all* cancer patients must face.

A detailed section on dealing with diagnosis and doctors will give you important guidelines to use for asking questions about your cancer, educating yourself about your particular diagnosis, and deciding how to discuss your condition with friends and family members. Finally, this chapter discusses treatments such as radiation and chemotherapy.

Being diagnosed with any kind of cancer is like suddenly landing in a foreign country. You quickly become aware of language barriers—everything is in Medicalspeak; cultural barriers—hospital life isn't like other environments you're used to; and a lack of comrades—you suddenly feel isolated and are surrounded by strangers. So, cancer patients usually go through a crash course on their particular kind of cancer. They get educated, they learn how to navigate and maximize hospital visits, and they ultimately discover parts of themselves they never knew existed. Let's get started so you can get on with treatment decisions and the rest of your life.

WHAT IS CANCER?

Cancer is the general term for abnormal growth of cells; a cluster of cells that go out of control and multiply. When the abnormal cell reproduces, it has the ability to invade, or metastasize to other parts of the body. The actual word *cancer* is Latin for crab. It was, in fact, the crablike appearance of advanced breast tumors that inspired the Roman physician Galen to name cancer *crab*. In Greek, "karkinos" originally meant "crab," too, which is how Hippocrates first identified and classified this illness 2,500 years ago.

Cancer was an extremely rare disease in the ancient world and is not mentioned at all in the Bible or the *Yellow Emperor's Classic of Internal Medicine,* the medicine book of old China. It began to be seen more extensively around the time of the Industrial Revolution, and by the start of this century, the annual mortality rate from cancer in the United States was about 4 percent.

Actually, the cancer cell itself is not dangerous (unlike bacteria or viruses), but its impact on the rest of your organs is. As it spreads into various parts of your body, it interferes with the jobs of regular cells, confuses other organs, and can wreak havoc on your system. It's basically a terrorist, hijacking organs and other cells. Cancer cells use the lymph system to get into the bloodstream and then travel throughout the body. These cells love organs that have multiple blood vessels and nutrients, such as bones, lungs, and brains—common sites to which cancer spreads.

Learning the Language

Cancer cells are divided into two groups: carcinoma and sarcoma. A carcinoma refers to cancerous cells made of epithelial cells, those that line various tissues. You'll find carcinomas in organs that tend to secrete something (milk, mucus, digestive juices, and so on). Common sites for carcinomas are breasts, lungs, and colons; common gynecological sites are the ovaries, cervix, and endometrium. Carcinomas account for 80 to 90 percent of all human cancers, and are generally slow growing. There is always a prefix attached to the word *carcinoma* that will tell you where the carcinoma is growing, and the kind of cells that are involved. An adenocarcinoma, for example, is a carcinoma made of glandular cells. When you just see the suffix *oma* by itself, it means benign. An adenoma refers to a clump of benign glandular cells; a fibroma refers to a clump of benign fibrous cells, and so on. When the cells are malignant, the word *carcinoma* is attached to the end, as in adenocarcinoma. It gets even more specific. You'll need to know where the adenocarcinoma itself originated. Think of it like this: "carcinoma" used by itself is as descriptive as saying "sweater." Adenocarcinoma is like saying "wool sweater." More specific descriptions can be "lambswool sweater" or "angora sweater." There can be other prefixes that are synonymous with saying "blue angora sweater." Other prefixes describe the shape of the cancer cell, like saying "V-necked, angora sweater." The point is you need not worry about a lengthy, unpronounceable name attached to your cancer; if a long prefix is attached to the word carcinoma, it's just describing it more accurately. There are literally hundreds of carcinomas, all described by a different combination of prefixes, identifying the parts of the bodies that are involved, the shape of the carcinomas, and so on. Carcinomas are sometimes named after the doctor who discovered them.

Sarcomas are cancerous cells made up of supporting connective tissue. Sarcomas are rare and account for only 2 percent of all human cancers but tend to be more aggressive than carcinomas. Again, the prefixes before the word tell you where the sarcoma is located, what it's made of, what shape it is, and so on. Sometimes sarcomas, too, are named after the doctors who discovered them. The suffix *oma* in Sarcomaspeak means benign, as in leiomyoma (which is the clinical term for a fibroid).

TABLE 10.1 **"Tumorspeak": Understanding What Your Doctor Is Trying to Tell You**

Tissue of Origin (where the cancer was born)	Benign Tumor (not cancerous)	Malignant Tumor (cancerous)
Epithelial		
surface epithelium	papilloma	carcinoma
epithelial lining of glands or ducts	adenoma	adenocarcinoma
Connective tissue and muscle		
fibrous tissue	fibroma	fibrosarcoma
cartilage	chondroma	chondrosarcoma
bone	osteoma	osteosarcoma
smooth muscle	leiomyoma	leiomyosarcoma
striated muscle	rhabdomyoma	rhabdomyosarcoma
Nerve tissue		
glial	glioma	
meninges	meningioma	meningeal sarcoma
retina	retinoblastoma	

Source: Adapted from Dorland's Medical Dictionary, 26th ed., by the Trustees of the University of Pennsylvania (Philadelphia: W.B. Saunders, 1981).

The difference between a carcinoma and a sarcoma is like the difference between a sweater and a boot; both are different things, but related. Nonetheless, they have different physical properties, are made of different materials, come in different colors, and so on. (You can also have a carcinosarcoma—a carcinoma and sarcoma all in one.)

In situ versus invasive

Regardless of whether you have a carcinoma or sarcoma of some kind, the most important words are *in situ* and *invasive*. In situ means "in one place." A carcinoma in situ means the carcinoma is confined to a specific area and has not spread. This is good news and means that your cancer is, by definition, non-invasive, and is in an early stage. Invasive carcinoma means that the cancer has spread to local tissue, surrounding tissue, lymph nodes, or other organs. This is not good news and means that your cancer is in a later stage. However, even though a cancer may be invasive and at a later stage, it can still be quite treatable.

Differentiated versus undifferentiated

Cancer cells are classified into two behavioral categories: differentiated and undifferentiated. These terms refer to the sophistication of the cancer cells. Differentiated cancer cells resemble the cells of their origin. A differentiated cancer cell that originates in the colon, for example, would look and act like a normal "colon" cell. In fact, these cancer cells might actually assist the other cells with routine functions. Because these cells spend some of their time assisting the body, they spend less time reproducing, and therefore take a lot longer to metastasize, or spread, to other parts of the body. Both differentiated and undifferentiated cancers are equally treatable; key factors are tumor size and lymph node status. Often, you won't find a purely differentiated cell. It may look just moderately abnormal. Because of this, there are subclassifications: moderately differentiated, well differentiated, or poorly differentiated. These classifications are known as the cells' *grading*. A high grade means that the cell is immature, poorly differentiated, and therefore faster growing; a low-grade cancer cell is mature, well differentiated, slow growing, and less aggressive. Remember, this is an extremely basic explanation of cell grading, which is based on far more complex criteria.

Undifferentiated cancer is made up of very primitive cells; these look wild and untamed, bearing little or no resemblance to the cells of origin. They don't assist the body at all, and are therefore able to spend all of their time reproducing. This is more dangerous because the cells may spread faster. There are cases, though, when undifferentiated cancer is not very aggressive, despite the fact that it's a more primitive cell. In these situations, it looks more wild than it behaves. This is often the case in breast cancers.

There are also mixes of these different cells; these affect the aggressiveness of the disease. For example, you can have mostly differentiated cells, mixed in with a few undifferentiated cells, or vice versa. Whatever is predominant will affect the behavior of the cancer; mostly differentiated cells will slow down whatever undifferentiated cells exist, while mostly undifferentiated cells will speed up whatever differentiated cells exist.

There are dozens of other cancer cell traits that will have direct bearing on how well they respond to treatment. For example, in breast cancer, many cancer cells respond to either estrogen or progesterone, and hence can be treated with hormone therapy in addition to other traditional methods. Pathologists can pinpoint where your cancer cells have invaded into surrounding tissue, and break down the metastasis into vascular invasion (cancer within a blood vessel) or lymphatic invasion (cancer within lymphatic vessels or lymph nodes); they can estimate how fast the cell is reproducing; and whether there are any dead cancer cells around, meaning that the cells are growing so fast that they've cut off their own blood supply and are leaving a dead cell trail (called *necrosis*). All of these factors are important and will affect your treatment and prognosis. Where the cancer is growing determines the kind of cancer cell you have. For example, stomach cancer will spread as stomach cancer cells. They won't suddenly turn into liver cancer cells as soon as they reach your liver, or lymphoma, when they reach your lymph nodes.

Designer Genes

It is now known that genetics plays a role in a variety of cancers, particularly colon cancer. People who have a family history of colon cancer are more likely to develop it as well. That's why it's important for your doctor to know whether any kind of cancer runs in your family. This has led researchers into trying to isolate specific oncogenes within our genetic makeup. The word *onco* means tumor; the field of oncology therefore means "tumorology."

One theory is that every individual has certain oncogenes that remain dormant in the body until an external agent turns them on (like a switch). Once turned on, the oncogene is responsible for transforming normal cells into abnormal cells. For example, if you carry the oncogene for breast cancer, many factors may trip its switch: poor diet, exposure to toxins, and so on. What trips your switch, however, may not trip your neighbor's cancer switch, which may be why some people get cancer, while others do not. So in this sense, while cancers are believed to be genetic, most scientists agree that external or environmental factors are responsible for triggering them.

Here's one way to think about it: we may all have some sort of weapon inside of us. Some of us have .38 caliber pistols; some of us have Uzis; some of us have cannons; and so on. But the cells that pull the trigger only do so when repeatedly provoked by outside forces, such as tobacco, X rays, excess estrogen, sunlight, radioactive fallout, or industrial agents. So while one cigarette may irritate your lung cells, twenty years of smoking may provide multiple "hits" to these cells that finally provoke them to pull the trigger.

Blood tests that detect various oncogenes are already being developed, and by the year 2000, screenings for a variety of oncogenes may be possible. People then could be treated or monitored long before their cancers would become life threatening. Certain blood tests now detect cancer trails (sheddings from cancer cells) in the bloodstream. These tests are currently being used to detect recurrences of certain cancers.

Cancer Culture

The adage "Keep your friends close and your enemies closer" is very applicable when it comes to understanding your cancer. You need to know the motives of your cancer so you can grasp the rationale of the various treatments you'll be offered.

Since cancer cells are living cells, it's in their nature to continue to live. So the first thing cancer cells do is grow. They'll simply begin growing where they first originated, be it the stomach or colon. The second thing cancer cells do is change. They mutate from the other cells that surround them. After they get to a certain age they want to move out and leave their original nest. So they spread out into surrounding fat and tissue.

A very crucial motive of the cancer cell is to eat. So the cancer cells send out protein messengers (called *tumor angiogenesis factors*), which create new blood vessels to feed them. If a cancer cell can manage these four basic functions, it will live, and the result will be a tumor. If any of these functions is stopped, the cancer will die. As you've guessed by now, treatments therefore attempt to interfere with these four functions; the goal is to stop the cells from growing, stop the cells from changing or mutating, stop the cells from spreading, or stop the cells from eating.

If the cancer continues to live, it will simply continue these same basic behaviors—it will grow bigger, change and mutate even more to trick the immune system, and spread out even more by bursting into surrounding structures and into the blood vessels. Finally, if the cells reach adulthood, they'll want to settle down and find a good home, preferably an organ with a lining in its blood vessels, such as liver, lungs, and bone. The cell attaches to these blood vessels, and passes through it into such an organ, and it will continue to make itself comfortable so it can reproduce more and more. This means setting itself up with a new blood supply to make the organ more conducive to its growth. And so it goes, until the cancer occupies every space in the body. The most important thing to remember is that none of this happens immediately; it can take years for this cancer cell to really spread.

TYPES OF GI CANCERS

There are several types of GI cancers you can develop, which are listed alphabetically below. The staging of your cancer (see below) will determine the kinds of treatments you'll be offered. Many GI cancers are treatable only when caught at an early stage. Because their symptoms are vague, many GI cancers go undiagnosed until the cancer is advanced. (Please review chapter 2, which discusses a thorough workup for general GI complaints. Some of those questions may be useful in catching an early-stage cancer.)

Anal Cancer
This accounts for about 2 percent of all cancers and is highly treatable. Roughly 90 percent of anal cancers are essentially skin

cancers that develop at the opening of the anus; they are often misdiagnosed as hemorrhoids. Anal cancer is associated with sexually transmitted diseases, and is more common in women, smokers, people who are immune suppressed, and in those who engage in anal sex. Surgery, radiation, and chemotherapy are all used to treat anal cancer, and the extent of these treatments depends on the size of the tumor and the stage of the cancer. If the lymph nodes are involved, surgery can be much more extensive as lymph nodes in the abdominal and pelvic region will be removed.

Colorectal Cancer (Cancer in the Colon and/or Rectum)

This accounts for roughly 13 percent of all cancers, and is considered the second leading cause of cancer deaths, next to lung cancer. Colorectal cancer develops from an earlier, benign growth, known as a polyp. Most colorectal cancers develop in glandular tissue but are considered very treatable when caught in an early stage. Ninety percent of all colon cancer is preventable through diet (see previous chapter), and because of active campaigns encouraging early detection (see chapters 6 and 9), many people will avoid a diagnosis of colorectal cancer. About 50 percent of all colon cancer is treated with surgery and adjuvant (preventive) chemotherapy and radiation (see below). When one to four lymph nodes are involved, survival rates are far higher than when four or more lymph nodes are involved.

Esophageal Cancer

When caught in the early stages, esophageal cancer is very treatable. The problem is that this cancer is often missed until it is in an advanced stage, when treatment options are limited. Thankfully, only about 2 percent of all cancers occur in the esophagus, and less than 10 percent of all GI cancers are esophageal. The symptoms of esophageal cancer are vague; they often include difficulty swallowing or frequent belching. That's why whenever you suffer from GI symptoms, it's especially important to have a thorough workup (see chapter 2). About 25 to 40 percent of esophageal cancers can be treated through surgery, but even then, the five-year survival rate hovers around 5 to 20 percent. These numbers are improving with better chemotherapy and radiation therapy. About 60 percent of esophageal cancers originate in the lining of the esophageal tube; 40 percent are glandular cancers. Poor diet is usually the culprit; it is seen in North America mostly in men over age sixty, smokers, drinkers, and in African Americans. (This may be purely socio-economic, however.) Men outnumber women by 3 to 1 when it comes to esophageal cancers; African Americans outnumber Caucasians by 3.5 to 1.

Gallbladder Cancer

This is an extremely rare kind of cancer, and when it rears its ugly head, it is usually in people with a history of gallstones (see chapter 7). This cancer is hardly ever detected in an early stage, unless it is found by sheer luck, when the gallbladder is being removed for the usual reasons (see chapter 7). So the treatment for this cancer depends on to where it has spread. The typical scenario is for this cancer to develop in an elderly woman with a history of gallbladder problems. Because of the age of most people with this type of cancer, treatment is also dependent on other health conditions. The survival rate is fairly dismal: less than 5 percent of those diagnosed will live for two years. But again, this is a very rare cancer—even in people with a history of gallbladder disease or surgery.

Liver Cancer

Liver cancer—that is, cancer originating in the liver, known as *primary liver cancer*—is a common cancer outside of North

America, but is fairly rare here. We hear a lot about liver cancer because this is the place where other cancers travel to, known as *metastatic disease*. For cancer to originate in the liver, some sort of toxin is usually the trigger, such as exposure to vinyl chloride or Thorostrast, or to aflatoxin, a fungus contaminant common in African soil. People with a history of hepatitis or cirrhosis of the liver (see chapter 7) are more prone to liver cancer, too. Studies show that steroid use, and possibly estrogen therapy, may put you at greater risk for liver cancer. Liver cancer also tends to develop more often in men than women; however, there is a rare type common in young women. Since your liver is responsible for removing toxins from the blood and metabolizing drugs, treating liver cancer with chemotherapy is difficult. Furthermore, the symptoms of liver cancer are vague, meaning that again, this cancer is usually advanced when discovered, and treatment is usually palliative rather than curative.

Pancreatic Cancer

This cancer is becoming much more common and is the sixth most common cause of cancer deaths. Ninety percent of pancreatic cancers are glandular, and it is more common in people over age forty, who have been exposed to petroleum compounds or solvents, people with a history of pancreatitis (see chapter 7), smokers, and people with diabetes. This is another one of those cancers rarely caught early enough to treat. It is usually found when it is in an advanced stage. A Stage I pancreatic cancer has a three-year survival rate of only 15 percent.

Small Intestinal Cancer

Cancer in the small intestine (see chapter 1), known as primary small intestine cancer, makes up just 1.5 percent of all GI cancers; esophageal cancer, still pretty rare, is much more common than this cancer. The reason small intestinal cancer is rare is because things move pretty quickly through this part of the intestine (see chapter 1), and there is less chance of cancer-causing agents "sitting around" in this region and having contact with membranes. They tend to either get lodged higher up (in the esophagus) or lower down (in the colon and/or rectum). Since the stool is still liquid at this stage, there is less possibility of the membranes becoming injured. The small intestine also secretes a large amount of liquids which can detoxify cancer-causing agents. When cancer in this region does develop, half the time it develops in glandular tissue. This cancer is more common in people over age sixty with a history of bowel disease (see chapter 6) or celiac disease (see chapter 2). People with a history of inflammation in that region could be more at risk for the development of a tumor. This type of cancer is treated with surgery and radiation, although radiation must be used sparingly, as the small intestine is highly sensitive to it. The five-year survival rates range between 20 and 50 percent, depending on the type of cancer and how advanced it is.

Stomach Cancer

This also is known as gastric cancer or gastric carcinoma. Stomach cancer can be treated and cured if it's caught in an early stage. But once again, because the symptoms are vague, 80 percent of the time it isn't discovered until it's in an advanced stage, which means that it has spread to nearby or distant organs (called *metastatic disease*). Stomach cancer is more common in people between age fifty and sixty, those living in lower socio-economic classes (diet related); and those exposed to certain industrial contaminants. People with reduced stomach acid (often due to previous ulcer surgery) or *H. pylori* infection (see chapter 3), smokers, drinkers, and curiously, men who live in colder climates are more at risk for stomach cancer, which most experts agree is generally preventable with good diet and life-style habits (see chapter 9). Surgery, radiation, and chemotherapy may all be part of the treatment for stomach cancer, but as this is usually advanced, the goal of therapy is largely palliative rather than curative.

Staging and Spreading

Four people can be diagnosed with the same kind of cancer, but each one will undergo completely different treatments, and face a different prognosis (predictions of how successful a treatment will be). This is because cancer is diagnosed at different stages. To complicate matters even more, each cancer has its own "personality." In other words, the same type and stage of cancer may behave differently in four different people. Most cancers have between four and five stage classifications that basically answer the question, "Where has it spread?" Depending on what stage your cancer is in, treatment and survival rates will vary.

Staging, in most cases, is determined by the size of your tumor, and whether the cancer has spread to lymph nodes or to distant or nearby organs. Usually, you won't know what stage the cancer is in until you have surgery to remove the initial malignant tumor. The following is a brief summary of staging for various GI cancers:

- **Anal cancer.** Stage 0 means the cancer is in situ, is non-invasive and microscopic, and hasn't spread below the membrane of the first layer of anal tissue. Stage I means a tumor less than 2 cm (1 inch) is present, but hasn't spread to lymph nodes or other organs. Stage II means the tumor is larger than 2 cm and may have spread into the muscle wall of the anus, but hasn't spread into lymph nodes or other organs. Stage IIIA means the cancer has invaded an adjacent organ, such as the vagina, prostate, or bone; Stage IIIB means the cancer has spread to the lymph nodes along the rectal wall or along the inner pelvic walls and/or groin. Stage IV means the cancer has spread to distant lymph nodes and organs, such as the lung or liver, which is metastatic disease.

- **Colon cancer.** Stage 0 means carcinoma in situ, which means the cancer has not spread beyond the first layer of colon tissue. Stage I means the cancer is confined to the lining or muscular wall of the colon. Stage II means the cancer has spread to adjacent organs, but has not spread to the lymph nodes. Stage III means the cancer has spread outside the intestine to one or more lymph nodes near the bowel. Stage IV means the cancer has spread beyond the colon to distant sites or organs, such as the lung or liver, which is metastatic disease.

- **Rectal cancer.** Stage 0 means the cancer is in situ and has not spread behind the membrane of the first layer of rectal tissue. Stage I means the cancer is confined to the lining or muscular wall of the rectum. Stage I means the cancer has penetrated all layers of the bowel wall, and may have extended to other tissues (uterus, ovaries, or prostate), but has not spread to the lymph nodes. Stage III is the same as Stage II, except now the cancer has spread to the lymph nodes. Stage IV means metastatic disease; the cancer has spread to nearby or distant organs.

- **Esophageal cancer.** Stage 0 is in situ; the cancer has not spread below the lining of the first layer of esophageal tissue. Stage I means the tumor is less than 5 cm, does not penetrate the muscular wall, and has not spread to lymph nodes or other organs. Stage II means the tumor is more than 5 cm and may involve the entire esophageal area, causing blockage; it may have spread to the lymph nodes but not yet to other organs. Stage III is what most North Americans have upon diagnosis. Here, the cancer has spread outside the esophagus, to the lymph nodes, but not yet to other organs. Stage IV is metastatic disease; the cancer has spread to other organs.

▣ **Gallbladder cancer.** Since this cancer is rarely caught in an early stage, the staging system used is simplified to three stages: localized, resectable (meaning the gallbladder can be removed); localized unresectable (meaning the gallbladder cannot be removed); and advanced disease, meaning metastatic disease, where the cancer has spread to distant organs.

▣ **Primary liver cancer.** As above, the staging system is simplified to localized, resectable (meaning the cancer can be removed); localized unresectable (meaning the cancer cannot be removed); and advanced disease, meaning metastatic disease, where the cancer has spread to distant organs.

▣ **Pancreatic cancer.** There is no Stage 0 here. Generally, any stage of pancreatic cancer means dismal survival rates (see above), but here is at least a description of where the cancer is. Stage I means the cancer is confined to the pancreas or has spread to the small intestine, the bile duct, or other tissues. Stage II means the cancer has spread to the stomach, spleen, or colon. Stage III means the cancer has spread to the lymph nodes. Stage IV means metastatic disease; the cancer has spread to distant organs and lymph nodes.

▣ **Small intestinal cancer.** Here, the staging system isn't used at all. Instead, the cancer is classified by cell type, which is a far more accurate way of determining how treatment will progress. Small intestinal cancer takes the form of adenocarcinoma (see above); leiomyosarcoma (see Table 10.1); and lymphoma (see above).

▣ **Stomach cancer.** Stage 0 means an in situ cancer; it has not spread beyond the top level of the stomach lining. Stage I means the cancer is confined to the stomach wall, and either no lymph nodes are involved (IA) or only local lymph nodes are involved (IB). Stage II is the same as Stage IB, except lymph nodes in the region around the stomach may be involved, too. Stage III is the same as Stage II, except now the cancer has spread to nearby tissues. Stage IV means metastatic disease; the cancer has spread to lymph nodes and to distant organs.

TNM

No, this is not a new cable channel, but a stage classification system currently used by pathologists to classify your cancer. TNM stands for Tumor, Node, Metastasis and uses a logical numbering system after each letter to describe the state of affairs in your body.

Very generally, T0 means your tumor was completely removed by your biopsy; T1 means the tumor is smallest, while T4 means the tumor is large and may have spread to other tissues. (T2 and T3 are therefore medium-sized tumors.)

N0 means "node negative"—no lymph nodes were involved. N1 through N3 indicate the lymph node involvement by degree; N3 is worse news than N1.

M0 means "no metastasis"; M1 means "yes, there's metastatis: the cancer has spread."

If you know the correct size of your tumor (which must be physically measured by a pathologist), and whether you're node-negative or node-positive (this information is determined after the pathology report, however), you can calculate your tumor and node class (your T and N class).

When it comes to the TNM staging system, an accurate tumor size should be shown in your pathology report. This is key. Unless the tumor is removed in one piece, it's difficult to accurately determine its size, which determines the staging. In addition, it's important that once the tumor is removed, it's measured accurately by the pathologist as well (something that isn't always done—particularly in tumors smaller than 1 cm).

DEALING WITH DIAGNOSIS . . . AND DOCTORS

When you're first told that you have cancer, you will be shocked. This can manifest into a variety of reactions from no response at all with some numbness to complete, high panic—your life may flash before your eyes, you can't think straight because your mind is racing in a hundred directions, and so on. Experts in the field of psycho-oncology, who specialize solely in dealing with patients' emotions and the many psychological issues of cancer diagnosis, classify the initial reaction of diagnosis as immobilization, shock, or high panic.

Another phrase used is "emotion versus no emotion." Denial of the diagnosis is also a common reaction (it can't be true; there's been a mistake; and so on), but this often takes the form of denying the seriousness of the diagnosis or its urgency (not to be confused with emergency).

What many top cancer specialists and cancer survivors stress is that a cancer diagnosis is *not* an emergency! You do not have to make decisions regarding your treatment in the next twenty-four hours or even the next week. It's taken a long time for your cancer to have reached the stage of discovery. As one specialist states, "Diagnosis does not mean that your cancer has suddenly developed, it simply means that you now know something more about your body than you did a day ago."

I promise—two weeks in the life of a cancer will not make any difference to your overall prognosis or survival. Take this time to absorb the information, educate yourself about your particular type of cancer (by reading detailed books about your specific cancer), and get a second opinion. In fact, many cancer centers today have a built-in second opinion structure, where members of a multidisciplinary team of specialists independently review each new diagnosis and, together, discuss their findings to make sure they all agree about the diagnosis, staging, and treatment recommendations.

Are You Sure?

If you're experiencing denial, which is a perfectly normal reaction to a cancer diagnosis, by all means, use that denial to learn more. Here's what you can ask your specialist as well as any consulting specialist (the second opinion doctor) to make sure there's no mistake, which will help you deal with the information more comfortably. I've taken the liberty of wording these questions in a way that you can use them as a script—in case you're struggling for your own words at the moment:

1. I've read that some tumors can look malignant but act benign and vice versa. Are you sure that my tumor doesn't fall into this category? (Note: indeed, the current classification system is flawed in that it can predict behavior of tumors based on certain biomarkers but it can't tell doctors everything there is to know about the biological makeup of each tumor. Similarly, you can predict how a baby will react to a loud noise, but you have no way of absolutely knowing until the actual occurrence.)

2. Are you basing this diagnosis solely on a single pathology report or have other specialists reviewed it? (Note: doctors are cautioned never to accept a single pathology report as the last word, and to never tell patients they have cancer based on solely written or oral reports.)

3. Have you discussed my current health status and family history with other oncologists thoroughly so you can recommend an appropriate therapy for me, personally?

4. Has the pathologist reviewed enough samples to make an accurate diagnosis?

5. Are you sure that the tissue samples the pathologist reviewed came from me?

6. Have you reviewed the pathology slides and report yourself? (This is key! Ask for a copy of the pathology report and ask your doctor to go over it with you and explain the report in language you can understand.)

7. How many cassettes (slides) were made from my biopsy? (Anything less than twenty cassettes per biopsy is a suspiciously low number. Twenty to thirty cassettes will ensure that nothing about the specimen was overlooked.)

8. Which "margins" were involved? (In the same way that a piece of paper has left, right, top, and bottom margins, so does a biopsy. Does the surgeon know if the cancer was closest to the nipple (medial), head (superior), side (lateral), feet (inferior), skin (anterior), or chest wall (posterior)?

9. (If you're more comfortable . . .) Can I request a second look at my tissue samples from a separate institution?

10. (If your doctor doesn't seem to know the answers to a lot of these questions . . .) I'd like to ask the pathologist some questions. Can you please give me his/her name?

Your specialist should not be at all annoyed at your questions. If she is, this is a bad sign, and you should try to go elsewhere. In fact, most cancer specialists are more concerned about the patients who don't ask questions (called *passive patients*). Unless you ask questions, your specialist has no way of knowing whether he has given you enough or appropriate information so that you can participate in treatment decisions.

Who Will Manage My Cancer Treatment?

Doctors work in teams to manage cancer therapy. This means that your primary care physician, surgeon (for surgery), gastroenterologist, radiation oncologist (in charge of radiation therapy), and medical oncologist (in charge of chemotherapy) are all involved with your treatment together. Either your primary care physician, gastroenterologist, or medical oncologist will act as your "project manager." The first thing you'll need to do after your cancer has been diagnosed is to get some answers directly from that doctor (most likely your gastroenterologist). The best way to get answers is to schedule a separate appointment with him or her, and use the entire appointment time for a question and answer period. Write all of your questions down ahead of time, and tape-record the answers so you can review them later either by yourself or with a supportive spouse (who should go with you to this appointment), partner, or friend. Often, when we're anxious, we don't hear correctly; we misconstrue facts and block out what we don't want to hear. That's why it's important to tape your doctor's answers. What should you ask? Obviously, questions will vary from person to person, but here are some general areas to get you started. While your doctor may not be able to answer all of the questions below, she can certainly direct you to someone who can answer what she cannot.

1. Find out where you can go for more information, and ask to be referred to a support group, a therapist, or a social worker who specializes in working with cancer patients.

2. Request the doctor to draw you a diagram of the cancerous organ or part, and shade in where the cancer is situated or has spread to. Visualizing the cancer makes it easy to understand.

3. Ask about the size of the tumor involved.

4. Ask if the entire tumor was removed when it was biopsied.

5. Ask whether the cancer is differentiated or undifferentiated. Your GI tract can be invaded by either kind of cancer cell.

6. What stage is the cancer in?

7. Does your hospital or treatment center have a multidisciplinary cancer team? This means that a number of cancer specialists—pathologists, surgeons, radiation therapists, and medical oncologists—discuss your case together and recommend treatment options.

8. Find out what treatment is being recommended and why.

9. Find out how the treatment will help, the risks/side effects associated with it, and the survival rates with successful treatment.

10. Find out where and when the treatments will take place, and how long they'll last. For example, if you're having radiation therapy, is your radiotherapy being done at an accredited facility?

11. What if you miss one treatment? Can you make it up?

12. What other health problems should you be on the lookout for during treatment?

13. How can you contact your managing doctor between visits?

14. Can you take other medications during treatments? How will the treatments affect other medications you're taking?

15. What about alcohol? Considering what you're going through, you might want a glass of wine or a shot of hard liquor occasionally. Is that okay?

16. If you're not given a very good prognosis, find out if you can participate in research studies or clinical trials using new drugs or therapies.

17. Find out what will happen to you if you choose not to undergo treatment. For example, if you have an advanced stage of cancer, are told that you will most likely not survive,

and chemotherapy treatment is not considered to be significantly useful, you may choose to fight the cancer with a gentler, more holistic approach, enjoying the time you do have left more fully. Many people do not regret this choice.

Second (and Third!) Opinions

When it comes to cancer, getting a second opinion means that you see two separate doctors about the same biopsy report to see if the diagnosis matches. You also see two separate doctors about treatment recommendations to see if the recommendations match. In the first scenario, if your tissue samples were carefully analyzed in the first place, you probably won't hear a different diagnosis, but when it comes to treatment recommendations, you very well may! Hearing different approaches will help you choose the therapy that's right for you.

Guidelines for seeking second opinions

It's usually routine to get a second opinion in a cancer diagnosis. But in case you don't feel allowed to go elsewhere, here are the general guidelines to follow. Answering "yes" to any of these questions means you're absolutely justified in getting another opinion:

1. Is the diagnosis uncertain? If your doctor isn't sure what your biopsy results mean, or what stage the cancer is in, you have every right to go elsewhere.
2. Is the diagnosis life threatening? In this case, hearing the same news from someone else may help you cope better with your cancer.
3. Is the treatment controversial, experimental, or risky? Since treatment guidelines for cancer change rapidly, what's experimental today may be standard therapy tomorrow. Nevertheless, if you're uncomfortable with recommended

treatment, perhaps another doctor can suggest a different approach.

4. Is the treatment not working? This is a question that may turn up in a later stage in the game. If you have a more advanced stage of cancer, for example, you may need to try another approach if you're not responding to a given therapy.

5. Are risky tests or procedures being recommended?

6. Do you want another approach? An eighty-year-old woman with heart disease and high blood pressure might be diagnosed with advanced colon cancer. She may die from heart disease or a stroke before she dies from colon cancer. As a result, her doctor may decide that she's too frail for surgery, chemotherapy, or radiotherapy, and opt to leave her alone. This woman may find this unacceptable and demand that her cancer be treated.

7. Are you uneasy with your current doctor? Always listen to that little voice in your head that says, "There's something that doesn't feel right, here!"

8. Is the doctor competent? If you have the slightest doubt about your doctor's ability, go somewhere else to either reaffirm your faith in him or her, or confirm your original suspicions.

How to Use a Specialist

Depending on where you live, you may not have the luxury of shopping for a specialist the way you do for a family doctor because you're usually only referred to one when you *need* one. And in smaller centers (particularly in Canada), there may not be any choice in specialists at all. Your main concern is getting better as soon as possible, and "getting in" to see another specialist in some places can take months—time you really can't afford when you're ill. But you have rights, and specialists, like any other doctors, have their rights as well. Because their time is valuable for both of you, here are some guidelines to follow to help you make maximum use of your specialist:

1. Tape-record your visit. Specialists often say a lot in a short time. When you're upset or overwhelmed by all of the information being hurled at you, you often don't hear what the specialist is saying. Tape-recording the visit is helpful because you can replay information when you're more relaxed, and better understand what you've been told.

2. Take along a family member or friend to this appointment. That way, you have support while you're there, and you can also discuss the information with someone who may have heard more because they are more objective.

3. When you have a lot of questions, make a list so you don't forget them. Take the list of questions with you, and tape-record the answers. The specialist has an obligation to answer all of your questions, and if he doesn't have time, there are some options. Give him your list and ask if he can address the questions in your next visit. If that's not possible, agree on a time when the specialist can call you at home and address them. As a last resort, ask if there is a resident studying with the specialist with whom you can arrange a question and answer session. (Usually, a resident is a "specialist in training" who can address your questions.)

4. Request literature or videos on your illness from the specialist, or the number of a support group, counselor/therapist, or organization you can call for more information.

5. Ask the specialist to draw you a diagram of your illness.

Dealing with the C Word

The most difficult part of a cancer diagnosis is dealing with the notion of actually having cancer. Your feelings about the diagnosis will obviously vary depending on the severity of your cancer and the statistical reality of survival. But even if you're assured repeatedly that your cancer is curable, the stigma of cancer is still there. To make matters worse, cancer patients often find that they spend most of their time reassuring other people that everything will be okay, particularly close family members and relatives. By the time they finish comforting others, and dispelling the third-party panic that results, they have very little energy left for themselves. Pity is another problem. When others are anxious about your condition and worry about how it will affect them or fear the same predicament, their response is pity. This emotion is characterized by an "I-would-hate-for-that-to-be-me" attitude. Nobody likes to be pitied. When people are supportive, however, their sympathy implies an "if-that-were-me-this-is-how-I'd-like-to-be-treated" attitude—a "do unto others" philosophy.

So what can you do to avoid the panic and pity of others? First, find out as much information as you can about your condition before you tell people other than close family members about your illness. For information and access to networks of other cancer patients, you can ask your own doctors, or contact cancer support groups or foundations in your area. Clinics and hospitals have social workers, psychologists, therapists, and support groups who exclusively work with cancer patients. Ask your doctor to refer you to one of these professionals. It's important to talk to someone who's had experience with other cancer patients, as well as to people who are going through, or have gone through, the same kind of cancer as you. That way, you won't feel so isolated and can keep things in perspective.

Or, you can turn to other support networks. For example, many corporations and businesses now offer a free program to their employees called the Employee Assistance Program. If you have access to this organization, you can speak to a qualified therapist in complete confidence, and at your own convenience, while your employer picks up the tab. These sessions are pre-paid, and the program is offered as a benefit and service to employees. If your company provides the Employee Assistance Program, brochures or posters are displayed on company bulletin boards with a 1-800 number. If you're not sure whether this is provided, ask your Human Resources Manager. Do take advantage of it if you can. Depending on your religious or community affiliations, there are also social service organizations that have social workers or therapists on hand; many people find turning to clergy comforting.

After you've done some of your own research, gathered some answers, or spoken to someone about your cancer, you will be better equipped to tell people about your condition.

Who can you tell?

What you say is as important as who you tell. That's why it's better to break the news about your condition when you're calmer and less frightened yourself. If you're married or in a relationship, your partner and children are usually the most obvious people on your list. I discuss this at greater length on pages 196–198. But there are usually other people you need to think about in addition to very close family members.

When you're ready, it's important to first tell people who are supportive. Figuring this out isn't always easy. Patient support experts recommend using "secret" rules. If you had an important secret to reveal about yourself, who would you tell? The answer should be someone you trust unconditionally. Second, it's important to ask yourself what the purpose in telling someone is, and what to expect his or her reaction to be. Asking yourself in advance may help prepare you for various responses.

Speaking from experience, I often say that cancer is like a wedding: It brings out the worst in some people and the best in others. For instance, people who you think are supportive friends can say the most terrible and inappropriate things. The same goes for family members. Meanwhile, the most caring and supportive people can pop out of the woodwork from the most unlikely places: acquaintances from work, public transit buddies, or fifth cousins twice removed who call you after they hear through the grapevine. But you'll most often find the best support is in a cancer support group, where you can talk and share with other people who are going through the same thing you are. Cancer survivors highly recommend this form of communication and support.

Making a list

After you've been diagnosed, make a list of who you must tell, and who you should tell. There's a difference. For example, if you have dependent children and/or a spouse, they must be told. Generally, your parents must be told (unless they're estranged or very old and the news would not do them any good). Anyone you live with or have an intimate relationship with must be told. Friends, business associates, and distant relatives, on the other hand, should be told, but it's not imperative.

Then, list on a separate sheet of paper who you want to tell. This category usually includes your real friends, or one best friend. Sometimes best friends are, in fact, family members—spouses, mothers, fathers, sisters, adult children (if you're middle aged, for example), aunts, or cousins. Often, best friends are outside the family. When this is the case, they're often more objective, and therefore more supportive.

It is this list that becomes your priority; the people you want to tell should be told before the people you must tell. You've chosen them because they're supportive and have proven themselves to you in the past. They will make you feel better, which will give you strength to tell the people who must know. Bad news is not the same as good news. Generally, you want to shout good news to the world, which means that the names on your "must," "should," and "want" lists differ drastically from the bad news lists!

When you're prepared to tackle your "want" list, make sure you choose your words carefully. For example, instead of saying, "I have cancer," begin with, "I have to have an operation." Then lead slowly into the reasons for the operation. That way, the information is presented in a logical sequence, rather than in an emotional sequence. Generally, the idea is to prevent someone else's panic—which will only make you feel more anxious. You can work on how to present your news by role-playing with your therapist. Or, if you have an open relationship with your doctor, you can discuss your condition and how to best present the news with him or her.

After you've told the people on your "want" list, you could ask them to be with you when you tell the people on your "must" list. That way, you have support should someone take the news badly.

To handle the "should" list, ask someone else to tell them— someone on your "must" or "want" list. That way, you don't have the extra burden of speaking to people you're not that close to or don't feel like telling yourself. As long as the people close to you know about your condition, you may wish to simply disregard the "should" list. Usually, people on this list are told out of politeness or a forced sense of loyalty. Unless there's a very good reason to tell them about your diagnosis, don't. To explain absences to business associates or co-workers, just tell them you're going to the doctor for some routine tests. That's all you have to say. Otherwise, rumors and through-the-grapevine gossip may result. (Unfortunately, other people's misfortunes are always considered the best "gossip.")

What if you don't want anyone to know? Depending on your situation, that's okay too (but it's a good idea to at least speak to a social worker). If you're older, are without a spouse, or have grown children, you may not have to say anything. But most of us don't have the luxury of complete privacy.

Telling small children

Small children are intuitive beings who will sense that something's wrong in the home. In fact, hiding the diagnosis from a small child is the worst thing you can do. Hiding a diagnosis may lead the child to conclude that she is the cause of your illness, for example. Cancer therapists recommend explaining the situation to a child in language she can understand, and if necessary, explaining or retelling over and over again. Younger children tend to repeatedly ask the same questions. This is their way of finding their bearings in a new situation. Hearing the same response helps to build consistency into a new reality.

The well partner or spouse should continue his or her routine with the children and watch for behavior changes. For example, young children may suddenly have difficulty at school, trouble sleeping, increased upset, and tantrumlike scenes. They may experience separation anxiety from the well or ill parent or create disturbing arts and crafts. A classic example of the latter is the child who suddenly draws pictures of monsters eating or attacking his ill parent.

Again, no matter how well you explain your illness, or how open you are with your child, exceptions apply, and some children will have more difficulty adjusting. You should seek out family and child counseling if you're worried about a child's behavior.

TREATMENT DECISIONS

Again, a diagnosis of cancer is not an emergency. It's important to understand all your treatment options before making your decision. Most GI cancers will involve some sort of surgery unless the cancer is in an advanced stage. Many of these cancers will also involve radiation or chemotherapy, often offered as a preventive measure after surgery.

Surgery

GI cancers often involve extensive, life-altering surgeries. Sometimes an ostomy is required (see chapter 6 and resource list). Sometimes dramatic changes to your diet and life-style habits will follow GI surgeries. The following are some general questions to ask before you consent to surgery.

1. If you're taking any prescription drug whatsoever, make sure you disclose the name of the drug and find out how long before the surgery you need to be off that drug. A class of drugs known as non-steroidal anti-inflammatories (NSAIDs) can be particularly dangerous.

2. The same goes for any over-the-counter drug, including ibuprofen, acetaminophen, and aspirin.

3. Ask about the likelihood of needing a blood transfusion. If there is a good chance of this, you may wish to consider what's called *autologous transfusion.* This may reduce the possibility of infection from a transfusion as well as the demand on the public blood supply. There is now a drug called recombinant human erythropoietin that is used to reduce the need for a blood transfusion. This is identical to your body's erthropoetin (the hormone that manufactures

red blood cells), and increases your red count prior to surgery. Your surgeon will fill you in on the details.

4. Find out how long you need to fast (if necessary) prior to your surgery. What foods should you stay away from before and after the procedure? Usually, you'll be told to have your last solids six hours prior to surgery and your last liquids three hours prior to surgery.

Other Treatments

There are a variety of other therapies, in addition to surgery, that you may be offered. The first question you'll need to ask is, "what's the benefit?" Often, there are no *tangible* benefits to these therapies, in the sense that you can look back a year from now and say, "Gee, I'm so glad I did that!" That's where playing the numbers game really comes in handy.

For example, if after your surgery for an in situ cancer, you have a very good chance of living cancer free for the rest of your life, chemotherapy may not raise the odds significantly at all. In this case, you'd be trading about six months of health and normal life for chemotherapy side effects, without getting a return on your investment. Is this a *benefit?* Many people would argue "No!" On the other hand, if you're not going to have peace of mind *unless* you have the chemotherapy, you might decide that, for you, the therapy is beneficial in that you can say, "I did everything I could to ensure my survival."

Weighing the benefits

By asking the following questions of yourself and your doctors, you should be able to arrive at a decision you can live with.

1. *How will treatment affect my day-to-day life?* Questions about fatigue, traveling to the treatment's location, sex life, child care, and so on are all valid. Find out!

2. *Will this treatment prolong my life (if so, by how much) or permanently eradicate the cancer?* In the final analysis, are you gaining years of life or "reassurance?" Know the true statistical benefits.

3. *How does my age affect the outcome of this treatment?*

4. *What are the short-term side effects of this treatment?* Nausea, vomiting, and hair loss are an example of "short-term" side effects.

5. *What are the long-term side effects of this treatment?* For women, premature ovarian failure, followed by menopause and permanent sterility, may be an example of a "long-term" side effect of chemotherapy (if you're premenopausal). Get all this information *up front* before you sign on the dotted line.

6. *Is this treatment covered by my insurer? If so, how will this treatment affect future coverage and my overall policy?* If you lose your insurance coverage over not-very-tangible benefits, you may want to reconsider. (This is not a concern if you live in Canada—as of 1999.)

7. *How will this treatment affect my immune system?* This is a crucial question. Chemotherapy, in particular, will suppress your immune system, leaving you vulnerable to infections and viruses you may never have had before.

8. *How will this treatment affect my job or future employment?* In essence, how much time will you need to take off work, and how much time can you *afford* to take off? Do you have long-term disability benefits? Can you take a leave of absence?

9. *Can you map out some "time lines" for the entire treatment process?* Take a daytimer or wall calendar into your doctor's office and literally plan what the timing of the various therapies will look like. Seeing it down on a calendar will help you decide whether it's feasible or not.

10. *What dietary changes should I be making to complement these treatments?* It's amazing how many people forget to ask this question, and how many doctors forget to tell patients about diet during various treatments. See chapter 9 for more information on nutritional guidelines and complementary medicine.

Radiation Therapy

Radiation therapy involves high-energy X rays or gamma rays (also referred to as "cobalt" radiation). X rays and gamma rays use photons (a photon has a different "dosage" of energy than light) to penetrate the skin. It is *not* chemotherapy. Therefore, your hair will not fall out unless your scalp is being radiated. Radiation treatment is very exact and directs radiation only at the areas where the cancer has spread.

The concept of radiation is very simple. Radiation alters the DNA of the cancer cell's nucleus (center) in the body cells it targets. The actual process, however, is a little more complex. First, you'll be referred to a radiation oncologist, an oncologist who specializes in radiation therapy. (This is *not* to be confused with a radiologist—a doctor who specializes in reading X rays and diagnostic test results.)

Radiation therapy is given over a long period of time rather than all at once, because the dose involves a fine balance: enough radiation to destroy cancer cells but not enough to destroy your healthy tissue, which is in a sense, "in the way" of the beam. Certain cancer cells are also more sensitive to radiation than others, just as some cockroaches respond to poison while others don't.

When radiation therapy is given as preventive therapy, to help prevent the cancer from recurring, the treatment scenario is usually one to three minutes of radiation every weekday from three and a half to six weeks. Most patients will have *external radiation* (meaning a beam aimed at the outside flesh). There are special cases, however, where internal radioactive implants are surgically placed directly inside a tumor.

Radiation therapy may also be used as a palliative measure in more advanced stages of cancer, not so much to cure the cancer, but to simply help relieve symptoms when a cancer has metastasized into other areas, such as lymph nodes or bones.

The dress rehearsal

Before you actually have your radiation treatments, you'll need to have a "simulation" exercise run first so the equipment, dosage, and targeted area can be precisely determined. You'll undergo a mock session with a "simulator" machine that looks like the actual radiation machine used in treatment—but isn't. Data is collected about your size, body shape, and the location and extent of the area that needs to be treated. The simulator also determines what kind of shieldings you'll need for the parts of your body *not* receiving radiation.

Getting tattooed

The radiation oncologist will either mark you with a "permanent" marker that wears off after a few weeks, or "tattoo" you by injecting tiny dots of special dye in precise areas (the size of a small freckle) he or she has first marked off in washable ink during your simulation. This dye will later be picked up by the radiation beam, which will use the tattoo as an exact target for a squared-off section, predetermined by the radiation oncologist. The tattoo is permanent, but fortunately is not very noticeable.

Once you're tattooed, you'll report a few days later to a radiation clinic, usually located in the hospital basement. Radiation clinics are situated in the basement because hospitals want to minimize the risk of radiation exposure to healthy people.

Reporting to a clinic in the bowels of a hospital may feel isolating and depressing. That's why it's important to bring someone along for support to the first few radiation sessions.

What happens during a radiotherapy session?

The radiation clinic will have a number of radiation therapists on staff who will operate the actual machinery, and administer your treatment. You'll go into a room that is darkened when treatment starts, and lie down on what looks like an examination table with a device overhead, which activates the beam. Then, you may be covered in lead blankets (this isn't always done), and only your targeted area will be exposed.

Dosage

The amount of external radiation you'll receive depends on the severity of your cancer. For example, you might only need thirty seconds of radiation every weekday for a month, while another person may require three minutes of radiation every day for six weeks. You'll receive a *total dose* of radiation measured in a unit called a "Gray," which is then divided by the number of treatments you have. This is called "fractionation." One Gray is equivalent to 100 rads.

Side effects

Although the procedure itself is painless, the aftereffects are not. Knowing this in advance won't alleviate the symptoms, but it may make them more understandable, and therefore more bearable. Although radiation therapy today delivers far less radiation to your tissues than that of even five years ago, you'll still have side effects from the treatment. For the first week of treatment, you probably won't feel much. By week two, the squared-off area that the beam targets will look and feel like a very bad sunburn. If you're fair-skinned, you'll probably have a worse reaction than people with darker pigmentation. Therefore, you'll need to treat your skin as though it *were* sunburnt: avoid sun, or cover up exposed skin; don't use any deodorants or perfumes; use cornstarch and lotions safe for sunburnt or baby skin. To help with the sunburn symptoms, ask the radiation oncologist or radiation therapist on staff for recommendations. Generally, diaper rash creams or sunburn creams safe for babies are quite good. Creams that contain lanolin will soften and moisturize your burnt areas (such as Nivea cream, for example). If a small area of skin actually peels, *before* it gets raw, 1 percent cortisone cream helps. For itchiness, cornstarch in a bath or applied topically with a towel and bandage is effective.

Radiation therapy to the GI region will cause a range of problems: nausea and/or vomiting; diarrhea; loss or appetite; and a range of upper GI symptoms, such as inflammation of the esophagus. *Make sure you find out exactly what to expect before your treatment begins so you can be prepared.*

Brachytherapy: "internal radiation"
This is sometimes given as a "booster" therapy after your external radiation therapy is over. Ultimately, it depends on your oncologist's treatment philosophy and the extent of your cancer.

Here, radiation oncologists plant a piece of radioactive material directly inside the tumor, or in the last known location of the tumor. In this case, a radioactive isotope (a radioactive element) such as radioactive iridium, gold, or cesium, is used to "blast" the tumor from the inside out, rather than outside in as external radiation does. In this case, tiny, hollow tubes are surgically implanted into the targeted area (the tubes are later removed), and the isotopes are placed into the tubes on your treatment days. Side effects of internal radiation therapy will vary depending on the area where isotopes are inserted. Skin irritations in the treated areas are not uncommon, accompanied by loss of energy and appetite. Side effects *greatly* depend on what's being inserted where. You'll need to discuss this in more detail with your radiation oncologist, and possibly a nuclear medicine specialist.

Chemotherapy

Chemotherapy was an accidental discovery that grew out of troops' exposure to mustard gas during both world wars. Although mustard gas wasn't officially used in World War II, it was during *this* war that the medicinal benefits of mustard gas became obvious. After a ship carrying the gas was bombed in an Italian harbor, survivors of the blast showed a dramatic drop in white blood cells—something that's bad news for healthy people, but good news for people with leukemia. The rest is history. Chemotherapy soon became standard treatment for leukemia, presenting the first possibilities for a cure. Within a couple of decades leukemia treatment formed the basis for treating other cancers: using poisonous agents to kill cancer cells.

Chemotherapy is a pretty universal experience for all cancer patients. In other words, whether you're having chemotherapy for stomach or colon cancer, the experience is the same. This treatment is by far the most miserable, and for many people, it makes the notion of having cancer a reality. In the past, chemotherapy was reserved for cases where surgery failed to treat the cancer. Today, even when there is no sign of cancer after surgery, chemotherapy is sometimes used as a preventative or prophylactic therapy, known as adjuvant chemotherapy.

What exactly is it?

Chemotherapy simply means treating some kind of medical condition with drugs. So technically, taking aspirin or an antibiotic are all forms of chemotherapy. When it comes to cancer, you are taking anti-cancer drugs. These drugs are designed to kill cancer cells. They interfere with the process of cell division or reproduction so that the cells can't divide and therefore die. But the drugs are not very selective and kill *healthy* cells that are also dividing, including hair cells and bone marrow cells.

Basically, the line between a therapeutic dosage and a toxic dosage is quite fine, and for this reason, only a highly experienced medical oncologist is qualified to manage your chemotherapy. Chemotherapy drugs can be administered orally or intravenously. You might be given just one kind of drug, or a combination of drugs. Combination drug therapy is often done because most chemotherapy drugs are not selective as far as cancer cells are concerned, so multiple drugs are used to overcome drug resistance.

Who is a chemo candidate?

If there is no evidence that your cancer has spread, and it was a small, localized, or in situ tumor, you won't be offered chemotherapy. You probably won't be offered chemotherapy if you're over age sixty-five unless your cancer is quite advanced. That's because chemotherapy is hard on the body, and generally not worth it for an older person unless there's a really high probability of the cancer recurring. Chemotherapy is recommended if you find yourself in one or more of the following scenarios:

1. Your cancer has spread to lymph nodes.
2. Your lymph nodes were not involved, but your tumor was large.
3. While there is no evidence the cancer has spread, there is concern that your cancer may recur.
4. Your cancer has spread to nearby or distant organs.

Common anti-cancer drugs

Once you enter the world of cancer drugs, you can quickly become overwhelmed by the various drug names. That's because one doctor may refer to a drug by its brand name, while another may use its generic name. For clarity, all of the generic names listed in this book appear first, while a common brand name is in brackets, as in ibuprofen (Advil) or acetaminophen (Tylenol). Also review Table 10.2.

Drugs you may come across in your treatment include doxorubicin (Adriamycin); cyclophosphamide (Cytoxan); fluorouracil (Adrucil), which has another generic name of 5-fluorouracil, nicknamed "5-FU"; methotrexate sodium (Methotrexate); and epirubicin hydrochloride (Pharmorubicin). Occasionally, vincristine sulfate (Oncovin) and prednisone (no specific brand name) are used as well.

When you're given these drugs in combination, the therapy is referred to by the acronym that forms when you put the generic names together. The only drug that is ever referred to by brand name within this acronym is Adriamycin. In other words, the "A" in *any* chemo acronym stands for Adriamycin. So for example, "AC" means your therapy is a combination of Adriamycin and cyclophosphamide. "CMF" means you're getting cyclophosphamide, methotrexate, and 5-FU. CAF would mean cyclophosphamide, Adriamycin, and 5-FU, while "CEF" refers to cyclophosphamide, epirubicin, and 5-FU.

Possible contraindications

These are very powerful drugs. As a result, you may not be able to take certain chemotherapy drugs if you have any "contraindicated" conditions, which may have nothing to do with your cancer.

TABLE 10.2 **Twenty-two Commonly Used Anti-cancer Drugs**

....

Aminoglutethimide, brand name Cytadren. An anti-hormonal agent, administered orally. Used to treat breast, prostate, and adrenal cancer. More common side effects include clumsiness, dizziness or lightheadedness when standing up, drowsiness, lack of energy, loss of appetite, skin rash or itching, nausea, and uncontrolled eye movements.

Androgens, generic names include fluoxymesterone, methyitestosterone, testosterone, testosterone cypionate, testosterone enanthate, and testosterone priopionate. More than forty brand names exist for the androgens, so check with your pharmacist, doctor, or nurse for the name of your drug. Androgens are male hormones, administered orally. Used to treat breast cancer in females, and for some other conditions. For females, the most common side effects, which should be reported to your doctor, include acne or oily skin, enlarged clitoris, hair loss, deepening of voice, irregular periods, and unnatural hair growth. For males, the most common side effects, which should be reported to your doctor, include acne, breast soreness, frequent erections, frequent urge to urinate, and increased breast size.

Cyclophosphamide, brand names include Cytoxan and Neosar. An alkylating agent, administered orally or by injection. Used to treat some types of cancer including Hodgkin's and non-Hodgkin's lymphoma, multiple myeloma, sarcomas, leukemia, neuroblastoma, breast, lung, testes, endometrium, mycosis fungoides cancer, and kidney disease. Side effects, which should be reported to your doctor, include dizziness, confusion or agitation, unusual fatigue, and missing menstrual periods. More common side effects include bone marrow suppression, hair loss, darkening of skin or fingernails, loss of appetite, nausea, and vomiting.

Doxorubicin, or Adriamycin PFS, Adriamycin RDF, or Rubex. An antitumor antibiotic, administered by injection. Used to treat some types of cancers including lung, breast, bladder, prostate, pancreas, stomach, ovary, thyroid, endometrium, sarcoma, leukemia, Hodgkin's and non-Hodgkin's lymphoma, mesothelioma myeloma, Wilms' tumor, and cancer of unknown primary site. Side effects, which should be reported to your doctor, include sores in mouth or on lips. Most common side effects include nausea and vomiting and loss of hair. Urine will turn red in color for one to two days after treatment.

Estradiol, or Estraderm. A hormonal agent, administered through patches placed on the skin. Provides additional hormones after certain types of surgery in females, and for other conditions. Side effects, which should be reported to your doctor, include breast pain, increased breast size, swelling of feet or

TABLE 10.2 (CONTINUED)

lower legs, and rapid weight gain. More common side effects include bloating of stomach, cramps, loss of appetite, nausea, skin irritation, and redness on site of patch.

Estrogens (IV). Generic names include chlorotrianisene, diethylstilbestrol, estradiol, estrogens, estrone, estropipate, ethinyl estradiol, and quinestrol. More than sixty brand names exist for estrogens—consult your pharmacist, doctor, or nurse for the name of your drug. A female hormone, administered by injection. Used to treat some cases of breast cancer in men or women, prostate cancer, to provide additional hormones after surgery, and for other conditions. Side effects, which should be reported to your doctor, include breast pain, increased breast size, and swelling of feet and lower legs. Another side effect for women who have not had their uterus removed and are taking estrogen in combination with the female hormone progestin is that they may begin having monthly vaginal bleeding similar to menstruation.

Estrogens (oral). More than sixty brand names and generic names. A female hormone, administered orally. Used to treat some cases of breast cancer in men or women, prostate cancer, to provide additional hormones after surgery, and for other conditions. Side effects are similar to estrogens in number 21, with the addition of nausea and vomiting, which are more common.

Fluorouracil, or Adrucil or 5-FU. An antimetabolite, administered by injection. Used to treat some types of cancer including breast, stomach, colon, liver, pancreas, ovarian, bladder, and prostate cancer. Can be used topically for skin cancer. Side effects, which should be reported to your doctor immediately, include diarrhea, heartburn, and sores in mouth and on lips. More common side effects include bone marrow suppression, loss of appetite, nausea and vomiting, skin rash or itching, loss of hair, and fatigue.

Goserelin, or Zoladex. A hormonal agent, administered by injection. Used in some cases of prostate cancer. More common side effects include decrease in sexual desire, impotence, and sudden sweating or hot flashes.

Leucovorin, or Wellcovorin, folinic acid, citrovorum factor, or leucovorin calcium. A protecting agent, administered orally or by injection. Used as an antidote to some anti-cancer drugs such as methotrexate, or a potentiating agent when used with fluorouracil. Also prevents or treats certain types of anemia. Side effects, which should be reported to your doctor immediately, include skin rash, hives, itching, and wheezing.

Leuprolide, or Lupron or Lupron Depot. A hormonal agent, administered by injection. Used to treat cancer of the prostate, and for other conditions. More

TABLE 10.2 (CONTINUED)

common side effects include decrease in sexual desire or impotence, nausea or vomiting, and sudden sweats or hot flashes.

Methotrexate, or Folex, Folex PFS, Mexate, Mexate-AQ, Rheumatrex, or amethopterin. An antimetabolite, administered orally or by injection. Used to treat some types of cancer including acute leukemia, sarcoma, choriocarcinoma, head and neck, breast, lung, stomach, esophagus, testes, lymphoma, and mycosis fungoides. Side effects, which should be reported to your doctor immediately, include black, tarry stools, bloody vomit, diarrhea, reddening of skin, sores in mouth or on lips, and stomach pain. Most common side effects include bone marrow suppression, nausea, and vomiting.

Mitomycin, or Mutamycin. An alkylating agent, administered by injection. Used to treat some types of cancers including colon, stomach, pancreas, esophagus, anus, breast, lung, cervix, and bladder cancer. Most common side effects include bone marrow suppression, nausea, vomiting, loss of appetite, and sometimes loss of hair.

Mitoxantrone, or Novantrone. An anti-tumor antibiotic, administered by injection. Used to treat some types of cancer including acute leukemia, breast, ovarian, and lymphomas. Side effects, which should be reported to your doctor immediately, include black, tarry stools, coughing, and shortness of breath. Another side effect, which should be reported to your doctor, is stomach pain. More common side effects include diarrhea, headaches, nausea, and vomiting.

Prednisone, or Apr-Prednisone, Deltasone, Liquid Pred, Meticorten, Orasone 1, Orasone 5, Orasone 10, Orasone 20, Orasone 50, Prednicen-M, Prednisone Intensol, Sterapred, Sterapred DS, or Winpred. An adrenocorticoid or hormonal agent which is administered orally. Used to treat acute and chronic lymphocytic leukemia, Hodgkin's and non-Hodgkin's lymphoma, myeloma, breast, and brain metastases, as well as some non-cancerous conditions. Common side effects include increased appetite, indigestion, nervousness, restlessness, and trouble sleeping. Side effects, which should be reported to your doctor with long-term use, include back or rib pain, bloody or black stools, chronic stomach pain or burning, puffiness in face, irregular heartbeats, menstrual problems, muscle cramps, pain, fatigue, reddish purple lines on skin, swelling of feet, thin or shiny skin, and rapid weight gain.

Progestins, or progestinal agents, known by several other names including Amen, Aygestin, Curretab, Cycrin, Delalutin, Depo-Provera, Duralutin, Femotrone, Gesterol L.A., Hylutin, Hyprogest, Hyproval P.A., Megace, Micronor, Norethisterone, Norlutate, Norlutin, Nor-QD, Ovrette, Pro-Depo, Prodrox, Progestaject, Progestilin, and Provera. A hormonal agent, administered

TABLE 10.2 (CONTINUED)

orally. Used to treat breast, prostate, uterine, and kidney cancer. These side effects are rare with this drug, but you should immediately get emergency help if you experience a sudden or severe headache, loss of coordination, loss or change in vision, shortness of breath or slurred speech, pains in chest, groin, or leg, unusual weakness, numbness, and pain in arm or leg. A more common side effect is a change in the menstrual cycle, which should be reported to your doctor. More common side effects include changes in appetite, changes in weight, swelling of ankles and feet, unusual tiredness, and weakness.

Tamoxifen, or Nolvadex, Novadex-D, or tamoxifen citrate. An anti-hormonal agent, administered orally. Used to treat some cases of breast cancer, endometrium, and ovarian cancer. More common side effects include hot flashes, nausea or vomiting, and weight gain.

Taxol, or Paclitaxel. An anti-neoplastic, administered by injection. Used to treat cancers such as cancer of the breast or ovary. Side effects, which should be reported to your doctor immediately, include cough or hoarseness, fever or chills, lower back or side pain, and painful or difficult urination. More common side effects, which should also be reported to your doctor, include flushing of face, shortness of breath, and skin rash or itching. Other common side effects your doctor will watch for include anemia and low white blood cell or platelet counts. Other more common side effects include diarrhea, nausea and vomiting, numbness, burning, tingling in hands or feet, and pain in joints or muscles such as arms or legs beginning two to three days after treatment, which can last as long as five days.

Testolactone, or Teslac. A hormonal agent, administered orally. Used to treat some cases of breast cancer in females. Infrequently causes diarrhea, loss of appetite, nausea or vomiting, pain in lower extremities, rash, and swelling or redness of tongue.

Thiotepa, or triethylenethiophosphoramide. An alkylating agent, administered by injection. Used to treat some types of cancer such as breast, bladder, ovarian, Hodgkin's disease, and bone marrow transplantation. Most common side effect is bone marrow suppression.

Vinblastine, or Velban, Velsar, or vinblastine sulfate. A plant alkaloid, administered by injection. Used to treat some types of cancer such as Hodgkin's disease, choriocarcinoma, testes, breast, lung, and Kaposi's sarcoma. Most common side effects include bone marrow suppression, nausea, vomiting, constipation, and sometimes loss of hair. Can cause burns if it leaks out of the vein.

TABLE 10.2 (CONTINUED)

Vincristine, or Oncovin, Vincasar PFS, Vincrez, or vincristine sulfate. A plant alkaloid, administered by injection. Used to treat some types of cancer including acute lymphocytic leukemia, Hodgkin's and non-Hodgkin's lymphoma, neuroblastoma, testes, sarcomas, lung, breast, cervical cancer, and Wilms' tumor. Side effects, which should be reported to your doctor, include blurred or double vision, constipation, difficulty walking, drooping eyelids, headache, jaw pain, joint pain, lower back or side pain, numbness or tingling in fingers and toes, pain in fingers and toes, pain in testicles, stomach cramps, swelling of feet or lower legs, and weakness. Can cause loss of hair.

Source: Drum, David, Making the Chemotherapy Decision, Los Angeles: Lowell House, 1996, 96–109.

Although medical oncologists take detailed medical histories so they can prescribe the chemotherapy regimen that best suits your physical condition, it's important to be aware of the following (and let your doctor know):

1. You cannot have chemotherapy if you're in early pregnancy, although most drugs can be administered after the first trimester. If there's a chance you might be pregnant, *get a pregnancy test first*, so you know.
2. You may not be able to have chemotherapy if you have chronic liver disease (especially if caused by alcoholism). You need a good, healthy liver to metabolize the drugs.
3. You may not be able to have certain drugs if you're already *immunodeficient* from HIV or a previous course of chemotherapy. You need to start with a healthy white blood cell count. (This is discussed later.)
4. Since certain chemotherapy drugs can induce lung disease, you shouldn't start chemotherapy if you have a pre-existing pulmonary disorder.

5. *Always* check with your medical oncologist before you take any over-the-counter or prescription medications. Painkillers that fall into the nonsteroidal anti-inflammatory (NSAIDs) or salicylates categories are especially dangerous. Certain antibiotics can reduce or increase the effectiveness of your chemotherapy.

6. You may not receive certain drugs if you have a pre-existing kidney disorder (although many of these drugs will affect your kidney function temporarily).

7. Let your doctor know about any bacterial, fungal, or viral infection. Insist on a full pelvic exam prior to chemotherapy so you can be screened for vaginal infections (yeast or bacterial vaginosis) as well as STDs (many are asymptomatic). Chicken pox or shingles (varicella) can be especially problematic with certain drugs, too. (Have you been exposed through your children, for example?)

8. If you're on hormone replacement therapy (HRT) or any kind of hormonal contraceptive, you *must* stop prior to beginning your chemotherapy.

9. If you have a pre-existing cardiac problem, you should not be on certain chemo drugs.

Dosage

Women who have been on birth control pills will be familiar with taking drugs in cycles. That's exactly how chemotherapy is administered. Some chemotherapy works on a twenty-one- or twenty-eight-day cycle, where various oral and intravenous drugs are administered for the first two weeks followed by a drug-free period. This is dubbed by insiders as the "two weeks on/two weeks off" cycle. Depending on the drugs used, you may be given a variety of drugs from days one to five, followed by a twenty-one-day rest period. Dosages really vary from person to person. They depend on your overall health prior to the chemo, the extent of your cancer, and a hundred other things. Many of the side effects discussed next can be signs of over- or underdosing; dosages need to be adjusted as your course of therapy continues.

How many weeks are we talking about?

Chemotherapy regimens last anywhere from three to six months. In more advanced cases of cancer, you'll have a course of chemotherapy, and then a "wait and see" period, sometimes followed by a repeat course of treatment.

In cases of recurrence, you may be cancer free for years and then need to repeat chemotherapy for a recurrence.

The general side effects

Each drug comes with its own list of potential side effects. For example, epirubicin will turn your urine red; doxirubicin can increase your risk of heart disease. Since space doesn't allow the listing of side effects for every conceivable drug or combination of chemotherapy drugs (this is enough information for a separate book), it's important to look up each specific drug you're taking in an appropriate reference. Pharmacists recommend getting information from the United States Pharmacopeia Drug Information (USP DI) or the American Society of Hospital Pharmacists book of drug information for consumers. Many pharmacies now offer extensive drug information for patients as an added service. Another option is to look up your drug in a pharmaceutical compendium, such as the *Physicians' Desk Reference* (in libraries) for the complete story; however, this information is very technical and may not be suitable for the layperson. I recommend getting this information prior to starting your drug therapy so you can review it with your doctor and be fully prepared.

There are general side effects common to all of the anti-cancer drugs. That's because no matter how balanced your chemother-apy dosage is, your healthy cells will be affected. Reactions vary from person to person, and there are certain medications, such as anti-nausea drugs (Zofran is a common one), for example, that are often added to your therapy to reduce the infamous vomiting and nausea.

Some of the more common reactions to chemotherapy include: tiredness, weakness, body aches, bloating and weight gain, night sweats, nausea, loss of appetite, and changes in your sense of taste and smell (you may notice a chemical odor all the time, for instance). It's not uncommon to have mouth sores, dry mouth, pink eye (conjunctivitis), allergy symptoms (watery eyes and runny nose), bleeding gums, and headaches, as well as diarrhea and con-stipation. Less common are tingling fingers and toes, and a loss of muscle strength. Some or all of the above may be mild, moderate, or severe, and you can take medications to relieve many of these symptoms.

Chemotherapy can also cause a chemically induced depres-sion (charmingly known as "chemo brain") and can induce dra-matic mood swings. If you're a menstruating woman, your peri-ods will become irregular or they may just stop altogether. This is because your ovaries begin to fail, which can cause you to go into surgical menopause, discussed later. In some cases, periods may return to normal after the treatment is over.

The most disturbing side effect is hair loss (clinically known as *alopecia*). It's important to be prepared for this, but there is also a possibility that your hair may *not* fall out. Talking to a counselor and sharing your feelings with other chemotherapy patients will help put this side effect into perspective. For some people, hair may thin gradually, while other people may find that they lose their hair suddenly. Still others may find that it comes out in clumps. Whatever the pattern, if you do lose your hair, you'll begin to notice it about three or four weeks into your treatment. You'll also lose all other hair on your body: pubic hair, leg hair, eyebrows, eyelashes, and so on.

One way to deal with this side effect is to find a good wig prior to your chemotherapy and have your hairdresser style it to your current hairstyle. That way, the wig won't look obvious, and your hair loss will not be as apparent. Many people simply adjust by wearing scarves, hats, or turbans.

Other side effects include a decrease in your blood platelets, which are responsible for blood clotting. You might find that you're bruising easily, bleed more when you're cut, or bleed suddenly out of your nose or even rectum. This will improve after your treatment, but report your bleeding episodes to your doctor so your dosage can be adjusted if necessary.

After your treatment is over, you'll start to slowly feel better. You'll gradually regain your usual energy and the depression will lift. Your hair will grow back in most cases, although it often grows back in a different texture (curly before; now straight or vice versa) and sometimes a different color (black before, now gray). You'll also shed the bloat and your complexion will return to normal. Food will taste right again, and you may crave foods you never liked in the past. You *will* be yourself once again.

Warning signs
If you experience any of the following symptoms, notify your doctor immediately. This is a sign that you may need to *stop* the chemotherapy *now*!

1. Severe diarrhea.
2. Severe stomach pains (sign of gastritis—inflammation of your stomach lining).

3. Dry cough (without sputum or mucus)—a sign of a possible lung infection.

4. An active infection or virus (flulike symptoms and fever should be reported).

5. Fever (especially if accompanied by a dry cough).

6. Shortness of breath.

7. Painful, frequent urination (symptoms of a urinary tract infection, which could be early signs of bladder inflammation).

Many of the "alarm symptoms" above are caused by too high a chemotherapy dosage. The general rule is to modify your dosage at the next cycle.

About your white blood cells . . .

All your blood cells and platelets are made inside the bone marrow. Normally, your bone marrow will be able to "recover" from the chemotherapy and get your counts back up to normal. But one sure warning sign that your chemotherapy may need to be delayed is a dangerously low white blood cell count (WBC). This is something you can't notice yourself (except flulike fatigue, which you wouldn't realize is a symptom), but will be apparent in your lab reports. In this case, your dosage is either adjusted or delayed until your WBC comes back up.

Sometimes you're given a white blood cell growth hormone, called *granulocyte cell stimulating factor* (GCSF). This stimulates your body to superproduce white blood cells like mad, raising your count dramatically from, say, a normal count of 10,000 up to 50,000, so your chemotherapy can be continued.

What happens in the case of very high dose chemotherapy regimens, necessary in certain cases of advanced cancer? Something known as a *stem cell transplant* is done prior to your next chemotherapy regimen.

In order to understand this, think about what happens in an in vitro fertilization procedure. In that scenario, a woman is given fertility drugs to help her ovaries grow eggs, which are then "rescued" from her ovaries and placed in a petri dish. Same thing here, except instead of fertility drugs, you're given GCFS to help grow white blood cell "eggs"—the stem cells! These stem cells are rescued through an intravenous procedure. Blood is taken out of one arm, passed back into another, and your stem cells are "caught" in between and saved in bags. After your high-dose chemotherapy, the stem cells are returned to you intravenously. Your white blood cell count will usually become almost totally depleted before your stem cells begin to produce them again. This will make you feel AWFUL! Generally, you'll feel like you were hit with a supermegaflu and will need to be kept in isolation during your chemo regimen. You'll also need to be careful about exposure to infections and bacteria, since you'll be completely immunosuppressed.

Long-term risks

Because chemotherapy blasts your white blood cells, it increases your risk of developing leukemia and possibly other kinds of cancers. This is, thankfully, a relatively low risk in relation to the benefits you receive from chemotherapy.

And because of the obvious potency of the drugs used, they can increase your risk of other diseases, such as heart disease and lung or liver disorders. Again, the benefits usually outweigh these risks, but you should discuss all potential long-term risks with your doctor prior to beginning your therapy.

Recurrent Disease

The ultimate question is, *Are you cured after all of these treatments?* The answer depends on the stage your cancer was in to begin with (see above).

If your cancer is treatable, it goes into remission, meaning that the cells stop growing, and what *was* there was removed or effectively killed. But cancer cells can start up again, and begin to grow at some future point. Sometimes the recurrence is local; sometimes the recurrence is elsewhere in your body (known as *metastatic disease*). Usually, the longer you go cancer free, the greater your chances are of being permanently cured. But there are people who see recurrences a decade after their first bout with cancer.

Recurrent disease means your cancer has come back (recurred) after it has been treated. It can recur in the same place as the original cancer or elsewhere in your body. In this case, you will need to repeat your therapy, or have more comprehensive treatment. This can involve more extensive surgery, chemotherapy (often for the first time), radiotherapy, immunotherapy, or a combination of treatments. It's also worthwhile to investigate the world of alternative or complementary therapies. Many studies show that complementary medicine can significantly affect survival rates for a range of cancers.

If this is the first paragraph you're reading, you've turned to a rather depressing chapter. I encourage you to go back one chapter, so you can understand how to prevent GI cancer and other problems. Regardless of what your GI "beef" is, it's all in here—from the upper GI tract to lower, from side to side, and everything in between. Don't forget to check the back of the book for a glossary of terms as well as resources for more information. As I say in this book's introduction, I hope this book helps each of you to stomach life on Earth a little better. I know writing it has settled my *own* stomach! Good luck and good health.

APPENDIX
Where to Go for More Information

Note: Because of the volatile nature of many health and non-profit organizations, some of the addresses and phone numbers below may have changed since this list was compiled. Many of these organizations have e-mail addresses, some of which are not yet made public. Please review "GI Online" at the end of this list.

United States

American Anorexia &
Bulimia Society (AABA)
293 Central Park West, #1R
New York, NY 10024
(212) 501-8351

Anorexia Nervosa and
Related Eating Disorders, Inc.
P. O. Box 5102
Eugene, OR 97405
(503) 344-1144

Celiac Sprue Association of
the United States of America
(CSAUSA)
P. O. Box 700
Omaha, NE 68131-0700
(402) 558-0600
Fax: (402) 558-1347
e-mail: celiacusa@aol.com

Crohn's & Colitis Foundation
of America, Inc.
386 Park Avenue South,
17th Floor
New York, NY 10016-8804
1-800-932-2423 or
(212) 685-3440

The Greater New York
Pull-thru Network
62 Edgewood Avenue
Wyckoff, NJ 07481
(201) 891-5977

National Association for
Anorexia Nervosa and
Associated Disorders
P. O. Box 7
Highland Park, IL 60035
(847) 831-3438

*National Digestive Diseases
Information Clearinghouse*
2 Information Way
Bethesda, MD 20892-3570

Overeaters Anonymous (OA)
World Services Offices
P. O. Box 44020
Rio Rancho, NM 87124

*Pediatric Crohn's & Colitis
Association, Inc.*
P. O. Box 188
Newton, MA 02168
(617) 244-6678

*Reach Out for Youth with
Ileitis and Colitis, Inc.*
15 Chemung Place
Jericho, NY 11753
(516) 822-8010

United Ostomy Association
36 Executive Park, Suite 120
Irvine, CA 92714
1-800-826-0826 or
(714) 660-8624

Hotlines

*American Dietetic Association and National Center for Nutrition
and Dietetics (NCND) Consumer Nutrition Hot Line:*
1-800-366-1655

Canada

*Canadian Celiac Disease
Association*
6519B Mississauga Road
Mississauga, Ontario
L5N 1A6
1-800-363-7296 or
(905) 567-7195

*Canadian Organic
Growers Inc.*
National Branch
Box 6408, Station J
Ottawa, Ontario K2A 3Y6

*Crohn's and Colitis
Foundation of Canada*
21 St. Clair Avenue East,
Suite 301
Toronto, Ontario M4T 1L9
1-800-387-1479 or
(416) 920-5035
Fax: (416) 929-0364
e-mail: ccfc@cycor.ca

National Institute of Nutrition
302-265 Carling Avenue
Ottawa, Ontario K1S 2E1
(613) 235-3355
Fax: (613) 235-7032

GI Online

Through the Internet, you can participate in newsgroups and bulletin boards (public forums) on digestive information. These can be accessed either through independent Internet providers or through an interactive computer service, such as CompuServe, Prodigy, or America Online (AOL).

Literature searches are great ways of getting specific information. Medline is the best search service for medical journal articles (many of which are extremely technical). Compuserve, Prodigy, or America Online all give you access to Medline. Medline is also available through many public and university libraries all over Canada.

Another way of accessing good information is through a Web browser, such as Netscape. By Web browsing, you can go to various sites in cyberspace to find information. When you don't know the World Wide Web (www) address, you can use a search engine such as Yahoo or Webcrawler to search for what you want by simply typing in your topic. The more specific you can be in your search, the better. A search engine is essentially an index to the Internet. When you go to a site, you can save or print the information. Flashing text (called hypertext) is a sign that you'll get more information when you click on it. This may even link you to other sites on the Internet. A good resource is *Internet for Dummies,* which will walk you through Internet access step-by-step.

GLOSSARY

abscess: An infected area of pus.

achalasia: Irregular muscle activity of the esophagus.

antacids: Medicines that relieve heartburn as well as peptic ulcer disease symptoms by neutralizing the stomach acid that rises into the esophagus.

anus: A muscular sphincter for the expulsion of waste.

appendicitis: Inflammation of the appendix.

appendix: Clinically known as the veriform or "wormlike" appendix, the appendix is attached to a section of the colon and is believed to have once played a role in digesting vegetation (such as tree bark or leaves). It now serves no known biological purpose.

autoimmune disease: A disease in which the immune system attacks the body's own tissues.

barium enema: A chalky solution inserted into the colon that shows up on X ray film.

Bernstein test: An "acid" test to determine whether symptoms are a result of contact between the esophageal lining and acid.

bile: Produced by the liver, bile is squeezed out of the gallbladder (where it is stored between meals) into the bile ducts when you eat and it helps absorb cholesterol.

candidiasis: Overgrowth of yeast or *Candida albicans*. Notorious for causing IBS symptoms.

celiac disease: An inherited disorder characterized by the inability to digest an extremely common food substance known as gluten.

cholecystectomy: A surgical procedure involving the removal of the gallbladder.

cholecystokinin (CCK): A digestive hormone that stimulates the pancreas to make enzymes and also causes the gallbladder to empty its bile.

chronic symptoms: Symptoms that are experienced on a regular basis for a long time.

chyme: Gastric secretions of the stomach which, when combined with mucus, hydrochloric acid, pepsin, and gastrin, serve to break down food.

cirrhosis: Inflammation of the liver due to viral infections, alcohol abuse, or toxins.

***Clostridium difficile* (*C. difficile*):** A common bacteria often caused by antibiotics, which kill off the bacteria that counteract *C. difficile*, allowing it to overgrow. *C. difficile* damages intestinal cells, causing diarrhea and inflammation of the colon (colitis).

colon: Major part of the large intestine; it extracts liquid from waste and turns it into recognizable stool.

colonoscopy: A procedure in which a long tube is inserted through the rectum in order to examine the colon and obtain a tissue sample.

colorectal cancer: Cancer of the colon and/or rectum.

colorectum: The lining of the tubing in the large intestine. The colorectum is made up mostly of muscle tissue, but contains some fat and lymph tissue.

continent ileostomy: A newer ostomy procedure that creates a waste pouch inside the intestinal wall.

corticosteroids: Powerful steroid drugs, such as hydrocortisone and prednisone, that control inflammation and suppress the immune system. They work by mimicking cortisol, an anti-inflammatory hormone made by the adrenal gland.

Crohn's disease: A disease that occurs when inflammation goes beyond the lining of the intestine into the actual walls of the intestine. Also known as ileitis or regional enteritis.

digestion: The process by which food is converted into the nutrients we need to live and the excess waste we don't need.

digestive hormones: Hormones that control the function of the digestive system and its secretions, released by the cells that line the stomach and small intestine.

digestive system: It is made up of two layers of muscle lined by cells and glands, which digest and absorb the nutrients and water from food. The muscles coordinate movement along the system.

diverticulosis: A condition arising from the development and inflammation of small, pea-sized sacs (called diverticuli) in the wall of the colon. They form in areas where the colon is weakened from bowel disease or from aging.

dysmotility: Impaired movement of some of the muscles in the GI tract.

dysphagia: Difficulty swallowing.

dysplasia: Occurs when the cells that line the colon become pre-cancerous as a result of ulcerative colitis.

early satiety: Feeling full after eating only a few bites.

endoscopy: A test for esophagitis caused by heartburn. A thin, lighted tube is passed down the throat and the esophagus.

esophageal manometry: A test that measures the motility of the esophagus.

esophagitis: An inflammation of the esophageal lining.

external hemorrhoid: Condition characterized by swelling or a hard lump around the rectum (due to a blood clot). Sometimes called a thrombosed external hemorrhoid.

extrinsic nerves: One of two sets of nerves that control the movement of the digestive system. Extrinsic nerves stem from the unconscious part of the brain or spinal cord. They produce the chemicals acetylcholine (which is what makes the muscles of the digestive tract squeeze the food through all that tubing, while forcing the stomach and the pancreas to squeeze out their juices) and adrenaline (which smoothes out the digestive tract muscles and decreases blood flow to the stomach and intestine).

fecal incontinence: The loss of control over one's bowel movements.

fistulas: "Ulcer tunnels" between tissues. Fistulas can develop around the bladder, rectum, anus, or vagina.

fundoplication: A surgical procedure that physically increases the pressure in the lower esophagus.

gallbladder disease: Occurs when gallstones (small stones inside the gallbladder) become large enough to obstruct the bile ducts.

gastrin: A digestive hormone that signals the stomach to produce acid, necessary for the breaking down of food. Gastrin also controls the normal growth of cells and tissue in the stomach lining, small intestine, and colon.

gastritis: Inflammation of the stomach lining.

gastroenterologist: A gastrointestinal or GI specialist.

gastroesophageal reflux disease (GERD): Also called hypomotility, this condition occurs as a result of dysmotility, and is characterized by a lack of sufficient contraction of the sphincter at the bottom of the esophagus, causing the stomach acid to back up.

Helicobacter pylori (*H. pylori*): Bacteria now believed to be the cause of ulcers. *H. pylori* lives in the stomach's mucus lining, causing it to slowly "wear out."

hemorrhoids: Swollen blood vessels or veins around the anus either inside (internal) or under the skin around it (external).

hepatitis: A viral infection causing an inflammation of the liver. There are three major kinds: hepatitis A, hepatitis B, and hepatitis C.

hernia: An organ that protrudes through its own cavity wall. GI hernias are the hiatal hernia (when a portion of the stomach pokes out into the natural gap between the diaphragm and the esophagus) and the inguinal or groin hernia (when a portion of the intestinal tract pokes through the groin).

H2 receptor antagonist: A medication that inhibits the stomach from secreting acid. Used mainly as a pain reliever rather than a drug that treats the underlying problem.

immunosuppressants (or immune modulator drugs): These drugs, such as azathioprine, are often used in cancer therapy. Since IBD is thought to be an autoimmune disease, suppressing the immune system has been shown to help "call off the attack" on the intestinal tissues.

inflammatory bowel disease (IBD): A serious, chronic condition occurring when one or more parts of the small or large intestine is inflamed, causing symptoms that range from unpleasant but manageable to severe and debilitating.

internal hemorrhoid: A hemorrhoid that protrudes through the rectum and hangs outside the body, also known as a protruding hemorrhoid.

intrinsic nerves: Found in the linings of the esophagus, stomach, small intestine, and colon, these nerves release a variety of substances every time food stretches out these organs. The substances either speed up or delay the movement of food through the digestive tract.

irritable bowel syndrome (IBS): Refers to unusual bowel patterns that alternate between diarrhea and constipation. Occurs when the nerve endings that line the bowel are too sensitive, and the nerves controlling the GI tract become overactive, making the bowel overly responsive or "irritable" to normal things, such as passing gas or fluid. Sometimes called functional bowel disorder.

lactose intolerance: A sensitivity to milk caused by an absence of the enzyme lactase, which breaks down the sugar lactose into glucose.

laparoscopy: Surgery done with a "keyhole" incision, with the aid of a telescopic instrument and video.

large intestine: The colon or large bowel. The large intestine stores waste products for a day or two before they are expelled from the body in the form of stools.

lepetomania: Excessive flatulence.

liver toxicity: This term is used in assessing risk factors from various medications. It refers to the risk of liver damage, also known as "drug-induced liver toxicity."

lower esophageal sphincter (LES): A crucial tunnel bridging the esophagus and the stomach, which acts as a ringlike valve that opens and closes, allowing food to pass.

lower GI tract: All of the digestive system below the small intestine.

macrophages: Special white blood cells that fight infection.

motility: The continuous movement characteristic of the process of gastric emptying, which is controlled by nerves, hormones, and muscles.

motility disorder: Occurs when the muscles in the esophagus and stomach region are not coordinating well enough to move food from point A to point B.

Mycobacterium paratuberculosis: A cattle bacteria being investigated as a possible cause of Crohn's disease.

non-ulcer dyspepsia (NUD): Discomfort in the upper GI tract not related to ulcer. NUD's symptoms may be indistinguishable from those of ulcers and heartburn.

nutrients: The by-products created when food and drink are broken down into their smallest parts to provide energy to our cells.

ostomy: An external pouch placed over the ileum's tip after a proctocolectomy, allowing waste to drain out. Combined, these procedures are known as an ileostomy.

pancreatitis: An inflammation of the pancreas that can lead to bleeding, tissue damage, infection, cysts, and even diabetes if the insulin-producing cells are damaged.

parotin: A hormone excreted by the parotid glands. Parotin helps maintain teeth, stimulates cell metabolism, and increases T-cell function in the immune system.

pathologist: A doctor who specializes in analyzing tissue specimens under a microscope.

peptic ulcer disease (PUD): A disease that causes a very specific, localized area of pain in the upper GI tract caused by a sore in the stomach lining.

peristalsis: The wavelike contraction of the muscles in the digestive tract that is triggered by swallowing food.

peritonitis: A condition occurring when the appendix becomes infected and inflamed and then bursts into the abdominal wall, causing the membrane lining the abdominal cavity (the peritoneum) to become inflamed.

polyps: Benign tumors in the colon or rectum.

proctocolectomy: Surgery used to treat ulcerative colitis, in which the entire colon and rectum are removed and the tip of the ileum (the lower small intestine) is pulled down and out of a neat, quarter-sized hole (called a stoma) made through the abdominal wall.

prokinetic drug: A drug that regulates the muscles in the GI tract by telling the brain to send the right "messages" to the muscles that control the GI tract. Prokinetic drugs help food get from the esophagus into the stomach, and then from the stomach into the small intestine. They do so by improving LES pressure and peristalsis, which gets rid of the acid in the esophagus and improves gastric emptying.

proton pump inhibitor: A strong acid-controlling drug such as lansoprazole or omeprazole.

ptyalin: An enzyme produced by the salivary glands.

rectum: Serves as a holding tank for the stool until it can be expelled from the body.

reflux: A fancy word for heartburn or acid indigestion, where semidigested food comes back up through the esophageal sphincter, causing a bitter taste in the mouth and a burning sensation in the esophagus. Reflux is usually a symptom of either GERD or ulcer.

regurgitation: The "coming back up" of semidigested food.

salicylates: A group of drugs that can reduce inflammation, especially in the colon.

scintigraphy: A gastric-emptying test that involves the eating of radioactive eggs that have been scrambled with technetium. A gamma counter then determines how quickly the scrambled eggs empty out of the stomach.

scleroderma: Hardening of the skin.

secretin: A digestive hormone that "kick-starts" all the pancreatic juices, which contain biocarbonate. Secretin also signals the stomach to produce pepsin (which breaks down protein) and the liver to produce bile (which breaks down fat).

sigmoidoscopy: A procedure involving the insertion of a short tube through the rectum with a lighted microscope on its end. Used to obtain a tissue sample.

small intestine: The midgut or small bowel. The small intestine can also be categorized as the duodenum, jejunum, and ileum.

sodium bicarbonate: An alkaline substance in the duodenum that neutralizes stomach acid.

stomach: An accordionlike bag of muscle and other tissue near the center of the abdomen just below the rib cage. The bag extends to accommodate food and shrinks when it is empty. The stomach itself is a "holding tank" for food until it can be distributed into more distant parts of the gastrointestinal tract.

stricture: The narrowing of portions of the intestine occurring in severe cases of Crohn's disease.

strictureplasty: A procedure that widens a stricture without removing any part of the bowel.

surgical resection: A procedure used to drain abscesses or remove various blockages that are a complication of Crohn's disease.

toxic megacolon: An enlargement and distention of the colon. Occurs in severe but rare cases of ulcerative colitis.

ulcer: Occurs when a small surface of an organ or tissue has "sloughed off," resulting in a sore.

ulcerative colitis: Occurs when inflammation and/or ulceration is confined to the inner lining of the colon (colitis) and rectum (proctitis).

upper GI series: A diagnostic test involving the taking of a series of images followed by a barium tracer to determine what's going on in the upper GI tract.

upper GI tract: All of the digestive system above the large intestine.

BIBLIOGRAPHY

Adamek, R. J., W. Opferkuch, and M. Wegener. "Modified short-term triple therapy—ranitidine, clarithromycin, and metronida-zole—for cure of *Helicobacter pylori* infection." *American Journal of Gastroenterology* 90, no. 1 (January 1995): 168–69.

Angier, Natalie. "How an opportunistic bacterium blitzes its way through the gut." *New York Times* (July 11, 1995).

Anvari, M., C. Allen, and A. Borm. "Laparoscopic Nissen fundoplication is a satisfactory alternative to long-term omeprazole therapy." *British Journal of Surgery* 82, no. 7 (July 1995): 938–42.

Aronsson. B., R. Mollby, and C. E. Nord. "Antimicrobial agents and *Clostridium difficile* in acute enteric disease: Epidemiologic data from Sweden, 1980–1982." *Journal of Infectious Diseases* 151 (1985): 476–81.

Arvanitakis, C., et al. "Cisapride and ranitidine in the treatment of gastro-oesophageal reflux disease—A comparative randomized double-blind trial." *Alimentary Pharmacological Therapeutics* 7 (1993): 635–41.

"Bacterial gastroenteritis is linked to the irritable bowel syndrome." *British Medical Journal* 314, no. 7083 (March 1997).

Bardhan, K. D., et al. "Lansoprazole versus ranitidine for the treatment of reflux oesophagitis. UK Lansoprazole Clinical Research Group." *Alimentary Pharmacological Therapeutics* 9, no. 2 (April 1995): 145–51.

———. "Rapid healing of gastric ulcers with lansoprazole." *Alimentary Pharmacological Therapeutics* 8, no. 2 (April 1994): 215–20.

Bartlett, J. G. "Epidemiology and clinical aspects of antibiotic-associated colitis." *Proceedings of the 2d International Symposium on Anaerobes,* June 22, 1985, Tokyo, Japan.

Beck, I. T., et al. Canadian consensus conference on the treatment of gastroesophageal reflux disease.

Bell, G. D., et al. "Effect of cisapride on relapse of esophagitis. A multinational, placebo-controlled trial in patients healed with an anti-secretory drug." *Digestive Diseases Science* 38, no. 3 (1993): 551–60.

Bender, B. S, et al. "Is *Clostridium difficile* endemic in chronic care facilities?" *Lancet* (July 5, 1986): 11–13.

Blum, A. L., and S. Huijghebaert. "Long-term treatment of gastro-esophageal reflux disease: Experience with cisapride." *Today's Therapeutic Trends* 11, no. 4 (1994): 219–47.

Bortolotti, M., et al. "Comparison between the effects of neostig-mine and ranitidine on interdigestive gastroduodenal motility of patients with gastroparesis." *Digestion* 56, no. 2 (1995): 96–99.

"Calories count in colon cancer risk." *American Journal of Epidemiology* 145 (1997): 199–210.

Carvalhinhos, A., et al. "Cisapride compared with ranitidine in the treatment of functional dyspepsia." *European Journal of Gastroenterology Hepatology* 7, no. 5 (May 1995): 411–17.

Castell, D. O. "Long-term management of GERD: The pill, the knife, or the endoscope?" *Gastrointestinal Endoscopy* 40, no. 2 (part 1) (March/April, 1994): 252–53.

———. "Introduction to pathophysiology of gastroesophageal reflux." From *Gastro-esophageal Reflux Disease.* Mount Kisco, N.Y.: Futura Publishing, 1985.

CCFA National Scientific Advisory Committee. *1997 Research Report*. Division of Digestive Diseases, University of North Carolina, Chapel Hill. Posted to: MedicineNet, Information Network, Inc., 1997.

Chal, K. L., J. H. Stacey, and G. E. Sacks. "The effect of ranitidine on symptom relief and quality of life of patients with gastrooesophageal reflux disease." *British Journal of Clinical Practice* 49, no. 2 (March/April 1995): 73–77.

Clostridium difficile. Document published by Maryland Department of Health and Mental Hygiene, Epidemiology and Disease Program, Licensure and Certification Programs, October 1989.

Cloud, M. L., and W. W. Offen. "Nizatidine versus placebo in gastro-oesophageal reflux disease: A 6-week, multicentre, randomised, double-blind comparison. Nizatidine Gastroesophageal Reflux Disease Study Group." *British Journal of Clinical Practice* Symposium Supplement 76 (November 1994): 11–19.

"Colitis responds to nicotine patch." *Annals of Internal Medicine* 126, no. 5 (1997): 364–71.

Collen, M. J., D. A. Johnson, and M. J. Sheridan. "Basal acid output and gastric acid hypersecretion in gastroesophageal reflux disease. Correlation with ranitidine therapy." *Digestive Diseases Science* 39, no. 2 (February 1994): 410–17.

Collen, M. J., and R. M. Strong. "Treatment of pyrosis does not insure adequate control of gastric acid reflux." *American Journal of Gastroenterology* 90, no. 4 (April 1995): 672–73.

Conference Reporter, Contemporary Issues in GI Motility Disorders. "Convincing clinical results with motility drugs force re-evaluation of the management of GERD." A special report from the Xth World Congress of Gastroenterology, October 2–7, 1994, Los Angeles, California.

Connelly, J. F. "Adjusting dosage intervals of intermittent intravenous ranitidine according to creatinine clearance: A cost-minimization analysis." *Hospital Pharmacotherapy* 29, no. 11 (November 1994): 992, 996–98, 1001.

"Constipation: Causes." Boston University Medical Center, 1996.

Costin, Carolyn. *The Eating Disorder Sourcebook.* Los Angeles: Lowell House, 1996.

Crohn's and Colitis Foundation of Canada. General patient information, 1995.

Dakkak, M., et al. "Comparing the efficacy of cisapride and ranitidine in oesophagitis: a double-blind, parallel group study in general practice." *British Journal of Clinical Practice* 48, no. 1 (January/February 1994): 10–14.

Dalton, H. R., and R. V. Heatley, eds. "Inflammatory bowel disease." From *Gastrointestinal and Hepatic Immunology.* Cambridge: Cambridge University Press, 1994.

Dashe, Alfred M. *The Man's Health Sourcebook.* Los Angeles: Lowell House, 1996.

de Boer, W., et al. "Effect of acid suppression on efficacy of treatment for *Helicobacter pylori* infection." *Lancet* 345, no. 8953 (April 1, 1995): 817–20.

Dehbashi, N. "Effect of triple therapy or amoxycillin plus omeprazole or amoxycillin plus tinidazole plus omeprazole on duodenal ulcer healing, eradication of *Helicobacter pylori*, and prevention of ulcer relapse over a 1-year follow-up period: A prospective, randomized, controlled study." *American Journal of Gastroenterology* 90, no. 9 (September 1995): 1419–23.

Dollinger, Malin, M.D., Ernest H. Rosenbaum, M.D., and Greg Cable. *Everyone's Guide to Cancer Therapy.* Toronto: Summerville House, 1998.

Duane, P. D., et al. "The relationship between nutritional status and serum soluble interleukin-2 receptor concentrations in patients with Crohn's disease treated with elemental diet." *Clinical Nutrition* 10 (1991): 222–27.

Dworkin, B. M., et al. "Open label study of long-term effectiveness of cisapride in patients with idiopathic gastroparesis." *Digestive Diseases Science* 7 (1994): 1395–98.

"Engineering a treatment for Crohn's disease." *Lancet* 349, no. 9051 (February 22, 1997).

Fanning, J., and R. D. Hilgers. "Ondansetron and metoclopramide fail to prevent vomiting secondary to ultra-high-dose cisplatin-carboplatin chemotherapy." *Obstetrics Gynecology* 83, no. 4 (April 1994): 601–4.

Fehr, H. F. "Risk factors, co-medication, and concomitant diseases: Their influence on the outcome of therapy with cisapride." *Scandinavian Journal of Gastroenterology* 28, suppl. 195 (1993): 40–46.

Fennerty, M. B. "*Helicobacter pylori.*" *Archives of Internal Medicine* 154 (1994): 721–27.

Fisher, R. S., and C. P. Ogorek. "Management of gastroesophageal reflux disease, part one: Pathogenesis, symptoms, and diagnosis." *Practice Gastroenterology* 18, no. 9 (1994): 21–22, 24–26, 32–35.

Fraser, R. J., et al. "Postprandial antropyloroduodenal motility and gastric emptying in gastroparesis—effects of cisapride." *Gut* 35, no. 2 (February 1994): 172–78.

Fudge, K. A., et al. "Change in prescribing patterns of intravenous histamine 2-receptor antagonists results in significant cost savings without adversely affecting patient care." *Annals of Pharmacotherapy* 27, no. 2 (February 1993): 232–37.

Fujimori, K., E. Suzuki, and M. Arakawa. "A case of bronchial asthma associated with reflux esophagitis, whose peak expiratory flow rate improved with omeprazole and cisapride." *Nippon Kyobu Shikkan Gakkai Zasshi* 32, no. 11 (November 1994): 1088–93.

Fumagalli, I., and B. Hammer. "Cisapride versus metoclopramide in the treatment of functional dyspepsia. A double-blind comparative trial." *Scandinavian Journal of Gastroenterology* 29, no. 1 (January 1994): 33–37.

Galmiche, J. P., et al. "Double-blind comparison of cisapride and cimetidine in treatment of reflux esophagitis." *Digestive Diseases Science* 35, no. 5 (1990): 649–55.

Geldof, H., B. Hazelhoff, and M. H. Otten. "Two different dose regimens of cisapride in the treatment of reflux oesophagitis: A double-blind comparison with ranitidine." *Alimentary Pharmacological Therapeutics* 7 (1993): 409–15.

Graham, K. S., et al. "Variability with omeprazole-amoxicillin combinations for treatment of *Helicobacter pylori* infection." *American Journal of Gastroenterology* 90, no. 5 (September 1995): 1415–18.

Halter, F., B. Miazza, and R. Brignoli. "Cisapride or cimetidine in the treatment of functional dyspepsia. Results of a double-blind, randomized, Swiss multicentre study." *Scandinavian Journal of Gastroenterology* 29, no. 7 (July 1994): 618–23.

Harries, A. D., V. A. Danis, and R. V. Heatley. "Influence of nutritional status on immune functions in patients with Crohn's disease." *Gut* 25 (1984): 465–72.

Hassall, E. "Wrap session: Is the Nissen slipping? Can medical treatment replace surgery for severe gastroesophageal reflux disease in children?" *American Journal of Gastroenterology* 90, no. 8 (August 1995): 1212–20.

Hausken, T., and A. Berstad. "Wide gastric antrum in patients with non-ulcer dyspepsia: Effect of cisapride." *Scandinavian Journal of Gastroenterology* 27 (1992): 427–32.

Heiselman, D. E., et al. "Randomized comparison of gastric pH control with intermittent and continuous intravenous infusion of famotidine in ICU patients." *American Journal of Gastroenterology* 90, no. 2 (February 1995): 277–79.

"*Helicobacter pylori*: A randomized trial employing 'optimal' dosing." *American Journal of Gastroenterology* 90, no. 9 (September 1995): 1407–10.

Hickner, J. M. "Ranitidine and GERD." *Journal of Family Practice* 41, no. 2 (August 1995): 186–87.

Hillman, A. L. "Economic analysis of alternative treatments for persistent gastro-oesophageal reflux disease." *Scandinavian Journal of Gastroenterology* Supplement 201 (1994): 98–102.

Hilts, Philip, "Risks of colon cancer." *New York Times* (April 24, 1997).

Hislop, Gregory T. "The role of nutrition in the prevention of cancer." *The Canadian Journal of CME* (March 1995): 111–18.

Holtmann, G., et al. "Dyspepsia in healthy blood donors. Pattern of symptoms and association with *Helicobacter pylori.*" *Digestive Diseases Science* 39, no. 5 (May 1994): 1090–98.

"IBS and Crohn's-Colitis FAQ." Edited and revised by Dr. Anthony Lembo, UCLA, 1996. Posted to the Internet: alt.support.crohns-colitis and alt.support.ibs. E-mail queries to: alembo@UCLA.edu or juniper@uiuc.edu.

"Irritable bowel syndrome." *Family Practice International* (September 15, 1996).

James, O. F., and K. S. Parry-Billings. "Comparison of omeprazole and histamine H2-receptor antagonists in the treatment of elderly and young patients with reflux oesophagitis." *Aging* 23, no. 2 (March 1994): 121–26.

Janisch, H. D., W. Huttemann, and M. H. Bouzo. "Cisapride versus ranitidine in the treatment of reflux esophagitis." *Hepato-Gastroenterology* 35 (1988): 125–27.

Jian, R., et al. "Symptomatic, radionuclide, and therapeutic assessment of chronic idiopathic dyspepsia: A double-blind placebo-controlled evaluation of cisapride." *Digestive Diseases Science* 5 (1989): 657–64.

Kellow, J. E., et al. "Efficacy of cisapride therapy in functional dyspepsia." *Alimentary Pharmacological Therapeutics* 9, no. 2 (April 1995): 153–60.

Kimmig, J. M. "Treatment and prevention of relapse of mild oesophagitis with omeprazole and cisapride: Comparison of two strategies." *Alimentary Pharmacological Therapeutics* 9, no. 3 (June 1995): 281–86.

Klinkenberg-Knol, E. C., et al. "Long-term treatment with omeprazole for refractory reflux esophagitis: Efficacy and safety." *Annals of Internal Medicine* 121, no. 3 (August 1, 1994): 161–67.

Labenz, J., F. Leverkus, and G. Borsch. "Omeprazole plus amoxicillin for cure of *Helicobacter pylori* infection. Factors influencing the treatment success." *Scandinavian Journal of Gastroenterelogy* 29, no. 12 (December 1995): 1070–75.

————, et al. "Effective treatment after failure of omeprazole plus amoxycillin to eradicate *Helicobacter pylori* infection in peptic ulcer disease." *Alimentary Pharmacological Therapeutics* 8, no. 3 (June 1994): 323–27.

Lepoutre, L., et al. "Healing of grade-II and III oesophagitis through motility stimulation with cisapride." *Digestion* 45 (1990): 109–14.

Lockhart, S. P. "Clinical review of lansoprazole." *British Journal of Clinical Practice* Symposium Supplement 75 (May/June 1994): 48–57.

Louw, J. A., et al. "*Helicobacter pylori* eradication in the African setting, with special reference to reinfection and duodenal ulcer recurrence." *Gut* 36, no. 4 (April 1995): 544–47.

Lux, G., et al. "The effect of cisapride and metoclopramide on human digestive and interdigestive antroduodenal motility." *Scandinavian Journal of Gastroenterology* 29, no. 12 (December 1994): 1105–10.

McCallum, R. W. "Cisapride for the treatment of nocturnal heartburn in patients with gastroesophageal reflux disease." *Today's Therapeutic Trends* 11, no. 4 (1994): 187–201.

McFarland, L. V., and W. E. Stamm. "Review of *Clostridium difficile*–associated diseases." *American Journal of Infectious Control* 14 (1986): 99–109.

Maleev, A., et al. "Cisapride and cimetidine in the treatment of erosive esophagitis," *Hepato-Gastroenterology* 37 (1990): 403–37.

Malkoff, M. D., et al. "Sinus arrest after administration of intravenous metoclopramide." *Annals of Pharmacotherapy* 29, no. 4 (April 1995): 381–83.

Markowsky, S. J., and M. L. Santeiro. "Automatic therapeutic substitution: Cost savings with intravenous push famotidine." *Annals of Pharmacotherapy* 29, no. 3 (March 1995): 316.

Marks, R. D., et al. "Omeprazole versus H2-receptor antagonists in treating patients with peptic stricture and esophagitis." *Gastroenterology* 106, no. 4 (April 1994): 907–15.

Mason, Michael. "Forget stress and spicy foods. The real culprit may be just a kiss away." *Health* (1994).

Mavromichalis, I., T. Zaramboukas, and M. M. Giala. "Migraine of gastrointestinal origin." *European Journal of Pediatrics* 154, no. 5 (May 1995): 406–10.

Merki, H. S., and C. H. Wilder-Smith. "Do continuous infusions of omeprazole and ranitidine retain their effect with prolonged dosing?" *Gastroenterology* 106, no. 1 (January 1994): 60–64.

National Digestive Diseases Information Clearinghouse (NDDIC), a service of the National Institute of Diabetes and Digestive and

Kidney Diseases, part of the National Institutes of Health, under the U.S. Public Health Service. Patient information, 1996. Licensed to Medical Strategies, Inc.

NIH consensus statement. "*Helicobacter pylori* in peptic ulcer disease." 12, no. 1 (1994): 1–15.

"Omeprazole versus ranitidine for prevention of relapse in reflux oesophagitis. A controlled double blind trial of their efficacy and safety." *Gut* 35, no. 5 (May 1994): 590–98.

"Open label study of long-term effectiveness of cisapride in patients with idiopathic gastroparesis." *Digestive Diseases Science* 39, no. 7 (July 1994): 1395–98.

Orihata, M., and S. K. Sarna. "Contractile mechanisms of action of gastroprokinetic agents: Cisapride, metoclopramide, and domperidone." *American Journal of Physiology* 266, no. 4 (April 1994): G665–76.

Orr, John. "Another man's poison." *Diabetes Dialogue* 43, no. 1 (Spring 1996).

Orr, William C. "The role of cisapride in the treatment of gastroesophageal reflux." In *Gastrointestinal Dysmotility: Focus on Cisapride*. R. C. Heading and J. D. Wood, eds. New York: Raven Press, 1992.

———. "Upper gastrointestinal motor functioning: A physiologic overview." *The Consultant Pharmacist*, Supplement A (1994): 4–13.

Park, K. N., J. S. Hahm, and H. J. Kim. "Pharmacological effects of metronidazole+tetracycline+bismuth subcitrate versus omeprazole+amoxycillin+bismuth subcitrate in *Helicobacter pylori*–

related gastritis and peptic ulcer disease." *European Journal* of *Gastroenterology Hepatology* 6, Supplement 1 (December 1994): S103–107.

Pedrazzoli, J., Jr., et al. "Triple therapy with sucralfate is not effective in eradicating *Helicobacter pylori* and does not reduce duodenal ulcer relapse rates." *American Journal of Gastroenterology* 89, no. 9 (September 1994): 1501–4.

Pipkin, G., and J. G. Mills. "Treatment of nonsteroidal anti-inflammatory drug-associated gastric and duodenal damage. Efficacy of antisecretory drugs and mucosal protective compounds." *Digestive Diseases* 13, Supplement 1 (January 1995): 75–88.

"Predictive factors of the long term outcome in gastro-oesophageal reflux disease: Six year follow up of 107 patients." *Gut* 35, no. 1 (January 1994): 8–14.

Rabeneck, L. "Long-term treatment of erosive esophagitis with omeprazole: Does it work?" *Gastroenterology* 108, no. 2 (February 1995): 613–14.

"Rapid eradication of *Helicobacter pylori* infection," *Alimentary Pharmacological Therapeutics* 9, no. 1 (February 1995): 41–46.

Reekie, W. D., and M. J. Buxton. Cost-effectiveness as a guide to pricing a new pharmaceutical product. *South African Medical Journal* 84, no. 7 (July 1994): 421–23.

"Return of Crohn's." *Lancet* 349, no. 9053 (March 8, 1997).

Rezende-Filho, J., et al. "Cisapride stimulates antral motility and decreases biliary reflux in patients with severe dyspepsia." *Digestive Diseases Science* 7 (1989): 1057–62.

Riezzo, G., et al. "Gastric emptying and myoelectrical activity in children with nonulcer dyspepsia. Effect of cisapride." *Digestive Diseases Science* 40, no. 7 (July 1995): 1428–34.

Rosenthal, M. Sara. *The Breast Sourcebook*. Los Angeles: Lowell House, 1997.

Schindlbeck, N. E., et al. "Empiric therapy for gastroesophageal reflux disease." *Archives of Internal Medicine* 155, no. 16 (September 11, 1995): 1808–12.

Shintani, S., et al. "Hyperventilation alternating with apnea in neuroleptic malignant syndrome associated with metoclopramide and cisapride." *Journal of Neurological Sciences* 28, no. 2 (February 1995): 232–33.

Sobhani, I, et al. "Platelet-activating factor stimulates gastric acid secretion in isolated rabbit gastric glands." *American Journal of Physiology* 268, no. 6, part 1 (June 1995): G889–94.

———. "Antibiotic versus maintenance therapy in the prevention of duodenal ulcer recurrence. Results of a multicentric double-blind randomized trial." *Gastroenterology Clinical Biology* 19, no. 3 (March 1995): 252–58.

Stubberod, A., et al. "The effect of cisapride and ranitidine as monotherapies and in combination in the treatment of uncomplicated gastric ulceration." *Scandinavian Journal of Gastroenterology* 30, no. 2 (February 1995): 106–10.

Sullivan, T. J., et al. "Short report: A comparative study of the interaction between antacid and H2-receptor antagonists." *Alimentary Pharmacological Therapeutics* 8, no. 2 (February 1994): 123–26.

Svendsen, L. B., et al. "Cimetidine as an adjuvant treatment in colorectal cancer. A double-blind, randomized pilot study." *Diseases of the Colon Rectum* 38, no. 5 (May 1995): 514–18.

"The truth about irritable bowel syndrome." Dr. Darren's Homepage. Queries addressed to DocDarren@aol.com.

Tofflemire, Jacqui. "Celiac Disease." *Diabetes Dialogue* 44, no. 1 (Spring 1997).

Toussaint, J., et al. "Healing and prevention of relapse of reflux by cisapride." *Gut* 32 (1991): 1280–85.

Tytgat, G. N. "Prognostic factors affecting the duration of remission of gastroesophageal reflux disease." *Journal of Drug Development* 5 Supplement 2 (1993): 21–25.

Tytgat, G. N., A. L. Blum, and M. Verlinden. "Prognostic factors for relapse and maintenance treatment with cisapride in gastro-oesophageal reflux disease." *Alimentary Pharmacological Therapeutics* 9, no. 3 (June 1995): 271–80.

"Ulcerative Colitis." National Institute of Diabetes and Digestive and Kidney Diseases, NIH Publication No. 95–1597 (April 1992).

Veldhuyzen van Zanten, S. J. O., et al. "*Helicobacter pylori* infection as a cause of gastritis, duodenal ulcer, gastric cancer and non-ulcer dyspepsia: A systematic overview." *Canadian Medical Association Journal* 150, no. 2 (January 15, 1994): 177–85.

Wagner, B., and M. Nagata. "Oral ranitidine as stress ulcer prophylaxis: Serum concentrations and cost comparisons." *Critical Care Medicine* 22, no. 1 (January 1994): 177–78.

Walan, A., and S. Eriksson. "Long-term consequences with regard to clinical outcome and cost-effectiveness of episodic treatment with omeprazole or ranitidine for healing of duodenal ulcer." *Scandinavian Journal of Gastroenterology* Supplement 201 (1994): 91–97.

Walsh, J. H., et al. "The treatment of *Helicobacter pylori* infection in the management of peptic ulcer disease." *New England Journal of Medicine* (October 12, 1995): 984–91.

"Washing hands reduces gastrointrointestinal ailments." *Family Medicine* 29, no. 5 (1997): 336–39.

Yousfi, M. M., et al. "Metronidazole, omeprazole and clarithromycin: An effective combination therapy for *Helicobacter pylori* infection." *Alimentary Pharmacological Therapeutics* 9, no. 2 (April 1995): 209–12.

―――. "Variability with omeprazole-amoxicillin combinations for treatment of *Helicobacter pylori* infection." *American Journal of Gastroenterology* 90, no. 9 (September 1995): 1415–18.

INDEX

rectal cancer. *See also* colorectal cancer
  staging and spreading, 183
rectum, removal of, 111

S

salicylates, 113
  for inflammatory bowel diseases,
    113
salmonella, 98
salt, 11
sarcomas, 171–172
scintigraphy, 36, 66–67
scrambled eggs test. *See* scintigraphy
screening
  for colon cancer, 116–117
  for *H. pylori,* 48, 53–54
  for ulcers, 48–49
second opinions, 186–187, 191–192
small intestine, 6–7
small intestine cancer, 180–181
  staging and spreading, 184
smells, 93
smoking, 14, 107, 166–167
sour stomach, 74. *See also* heartburn
Steingraber, Sandra, 157
stomach cancer, 52, 181
  staging and spreading, 184–185
stomach lining, breakdown of,
    43–45
stomach ulcers, 45, 47
stress, 43, 45, 46, 104
  bowel problems and, 104
support groups, 189, 194, 195
surgery, 111–113
  bowel transplants, 113
  for cancer, 199–202
  colectomy, 111–113
  gallbladder, 125–126
swallowing food, 4–5
swallowing medicines, 86
symptoms, gastrointestinal
  for alarm, 27–28
  despite treatment, 28
  what relieves, 30–31

T

tests, diagnostic, 34–36
thrush, oral, 147
thyroid disease, 145–146
Thyroid Sourcebook, The (Rosenthal),
    146
TNM staging system of cancer
    classification, 185
transfatty acids, 156
transplants, bowel, 113
tumor angiogenesis factors, 176–177
tumors, 171. *See also* cancers

U

ulcerative colitis, 105–111, 109–110.
    See also inflammatory bowel
    disease (IBS) *headings*
ulcers, 39–57. See also *Helicobacter
    pylori*
  duodenal, 43
  as emergencies, 49–50
  myths about, 45–48
  shapes and sizes, 41–42
  symptoms, 42–43
  types of, 39
U.S. Department of Agriculture,
    155, 158

V

viruses, 97
  cytomegalovirus infection, 151
  and liver, 16–168
vitamins, 11, 164–165
vomiting, self-induced, 138

W

washing hands, 166–168
wasting, 148–149
water and salt, 11
weight loss, and HIV, 148
wellness, and diet, 153–168
women
  digestion and female disorders, 15
  disorders of, 139–144
  irritable bowel syndrome and,
    104–105

3327